Diabetes Health Care

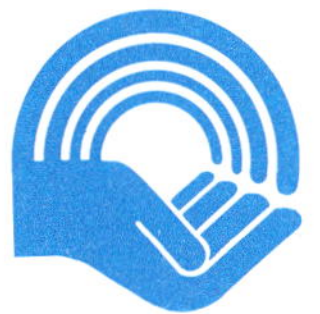

A Servier Service to Diabetes

Diabetes Health Care

A guide to the provision of health care services

R.D. HILL FRCP
Consultant physician
Poole General Hospital, Poole, Dorset

London
CHAPMAN AND HALL

This book is dedicated to the Family Doctors, Ophthalmic Medical Practitioners, and Ophthalmic Opticians, without whom the Community Care Service for Diabetics in the Poole area would not exist.

First published in 1987 by Chapman and Hall Ltd
11 New Fetter Lane, London EC4P 4EE

Printed in Great Britain at the University Press, Cambridge

ISBN 0 412 27330 6

British Library Cataloguing in Publication Data

Hill, R.D. (Ronald David)
Diabetes health care: a guide to the provision of health care services.
1. Diabetes — Services for — Great Britain
2. Medical care — Great Britain
I. Title
362.1′96462′00941 RC660

ISBN 0-412-27330-6

Contents

Acknowledgements

I extend my thanks to all those who have helped and supported the preparation of this text. In particular, Mrs Judy French and Mrs Val McBride for typing and constantly revising the script.

I am also grateful for the collaboration of my colleagues in preparing certain chapters of the book. In particular I thank Dr C. Upton, Dr R. Sadler, Dr Anne Gee and Dr R. Prior for their help in preparing Chapter 13. My thanks are also due to Mr C. Stiles (District Chiropodist), and to Susan Taylor and Vanessa Robson, (Chiropidists), and to Mr Frank Tovey (Consultant Surgeon) for their considerable help in preparing Chapter 11.

My thanks are also due to Dr Wendy Gatling, Novo Research Fellow, who has been most helpful in reading and correcting the text, and to Mr Andrew Barnett and Mr Barry Jenning, Poole General Hospital Photographers who have kindly prepared the photographic material. Mr Peter Barry, Consultant Ophthalmic Surgeon, Royal Victoria Eye Hospital, Dublin, kindly supplied plate 17.

I also thank the Editor of *Practical Diabetes* for allowing me to reproduce data in Chapter 14, previously published in *Practical Diabetes*.

I am grateful to the Ames Division of the Miles Corporation, and Servier Laboratories Limited for their support in providing illustrations for the text.

Finally I would like to thank my long-suffering wife, Juliet, for not only reading and correcting the text but also for her continued support through difficult times during the last 30 years.

Preface

This book is not intended simply as an educational aid for the Diabetic Health Care Team. It is also intended to broaden the horizons of the team as a whole.

I can expect to teach the diabetologist little diabetology but I hope to put in perspective his or her part in the team's activities. It is no longer enough for the consultant diabetologist just to run a diabetic clinic.

I hope that the family doctor will find the text useful not only as an aid to the management of diabetes but also to allow him to see how much is involved in diabetic care. If the large work load is to be coped with efficiently and effectively some form of integrated shared care is essential. The family doctors must be aware of the part played by other members of the diabetic health care team.

Consultant ophthalmologists may also be interested to see how an integrated service can be developed. The ophthalmic optician can play a truly significant role in diabetic health care and the text hopefully will be useful in providing essential and background information on diabetes and the diabetic service.

Dietitians now play an important part in the management of diabetes. It is often forgotten that this intelligent group of workers need more than simple instruction on what is the current fashion in dietary advice for the diabetic. If the dietitians are to play a full part in diabetic education then horizons must be broadened to encompass other aspects of diabetic care. Hopefully dietitians will find the text useful in providing both background and detailed information.

Nurses now play an increasingly important role in diabetic care particularly with respect to diabetic education. The specialist ward sister and specialist nurse (diabetic liaison sister) now require more detailed information on diabetes and must be thoroughly aware of the aims and functions of the whole health care team.

With an ageing population the chiropodist plays an important part in combating the ravages of peripheral vascular disease and neuropathy. However, the chiropodist cannot operate in isolation and must be integrated into the team as a whole.

Many other workers are involved in conveying health care to the diabetic. Some may find chapters of interest, and a brief glossary is provided to help those not medically qualified.

The great danger in such a venture as this is that in trying to be all things to all men the text will be nothing for everyone. The course between Scylla and Charybdis is a difficult one to steer. I can only hope that to some extent the voyage is successful.

R.D.Hill
Poole, 1987

Foreword

I have known Dr Ronald Hill since his student days at Guy's Hospital Medical School. When I first heard of his plans to develop a system of diabetic health care based with the general practitioners in the community, rather than simply on the diabetic clinics, I realized at once that his careful clinical approach and his interest in education and training both the medical profession and the patients themselves were being expressed again. I knew he would lay meticulously careful plans, carry them out slowly where necessary but always properly, reaching for the high standards worthy of emulation elsewhere in the NHS, and this book is confirmation of Ron Hill's personal achievement in the field where he is a pioneer.

He sets out for us excellent examples, explanations and model answers to the many problems involved in the safe care of the diabetic patient, not just in the clinical practice, but where the patient lives and works. He covers the whole ground, from the basis of diagnosing diabetes, to establishing control and treatment, to following the risks and needs of diabetic complications in the patients' eyes, kidneys, nerves and cardiovascular system. He shows how he organized, (and how you can do the same,) the community care services to humanize the management of a potentially damaging, certainly disabling, unremitting chronic disease. He shows what skills, patience and dedication will be required from us all, the diabetics and their families, and the health workers to whom Ron Hill has dedicated his book.

I wish the author, his ideas and the messages of this book a wide audience and proper appreciation.

Finally, please note well that the health care principles involved in this pioneer work for diabetics can now be applied to other chronic illnesses, where the patients' own actions can help or hinder progress in the application of science and biomedical technology.

Professor Sir John Butterfield
Cambridge, 1987

· One ·

An overview of diabetes mellitus

1.1 INTRODUCTION

This chapter is meant to be an overview of the subject. In-depth treatment is not intended. Certain aspects of diabetes are amplified in later chapters, and the reader is advised on further reading at the end of the chapter.

1.2 DEFINITION OF DIABETES MELLITUS

Diabetes mellitus is not a single disease but a group of diseases. The *sine qua non* of diabetes mellitus is abnormal blood glucose homeostasis which results in blood glucose values above the accepted normal range. However, how 'abnormal' is above 'normal'? The answer to this question is easy at the higher end of the scale of blood glucose values found in overt disease, but what of those blood glucose values that approach normality? Using a standardized carbohydrate stress test (the glucose tolerance test, or GTT) it has been shown that the glucose homeostatic mechanism varies with age, sex, time within the menstrual cycle and even with the time of day. In order to remove a little of the uncertainty from the diagnosis at the lower end of the scale a standardized stress test with normal values has been defined by the World Health Organization. A full GTT is rarely if ever necessary to define the diabetic state. The modified (2 point) GTT is all that is necessary if the diagnosis is in doubt. The conditions laid down for the modified GTT are:

1. Overnight (6–8 hours) fast.
2. Patient at rest – not smoking.
3. Fasting blood glucose (FBG).
4. Glucose load : 1.75 g/kg in children, 75 g in adult in 250–350 ml water drunk over 10 minute period.
5. Blood glucose 2 hours after glucose load.
6. Specific enzymatic glucose assay.

Table 1.1 Diagnostic values for oral glucose tolerance test under standard conditions. Results are given in mmol/l (g/l in parentheses)

	Glucose concentration		
	Venous whole blood	*Capillary whole blood*	*Venous plasma*
	Diabetes mellitus		
Fasting	≥7.0 (1.2)	≥7.0 (1.2)	≥8.0 (1.4)
and/or			
2 hours after glucose load	≥10.0 (1.8)	≥11.0 (2.0)	≥11.0 (2.0)
	Impaired glucose tolerance		
Fasting	≥7.0 (1.2)	≥7.0 (1.2)	≥8.0 (1.4)
and			
2 hours after glucose load	≥7.0<10.0 (1.2–1.8)	≥8.0<11.0 (1.4–2.0)	≥8.0<11.0 (1.4–2.0)

Source: WHO Expert Committee on Diabetes Mellitus (1980) *2nd Report*, Technical Report Series 646. WHO, Geneva.

1.3 WHO CRITERIA FOR THE INTERPRETATION OF THE GLUCOSE TOLERANCE TEST

The conditions for the performance of a GTT as laid down immediately above must be satisfied. In the modified GTT blood sampling is done in the fasting state and 2 hours after the glucose load. The precise interpretation of blood glucose concentrations found will depend on whether the specimens are venous, or capillary whole blood or venous plasma (Table 1.1). Glucose concentrations that reach or exceed the values shown indicate, by definition, that the patient has diabetes mellitus. A fasting blood glucose exceeding the values given should not be accepted as diagnostic unless the 2-hour value is diagnostic.

Those patients showing an abnormal response but who do not reach the diagnostic criteria for diabetes mellitus are said to have carbohydrate intolerance or impaired glucose tolerance.

NB. The glucose concentration measured in the GTT must be performed by a laboratory and reliance must not be made on blood test stix even with a meter. As indicated in section 1.4 the diagnosis has important implications and there must be no error in glucose measurement.

1.4 IN PRACTICE – ESTABLISHING THE DIAGNOSIS

What does this mean in practice? To establish the diagnosis of diabetes mellitus a blood glucose 2 hours after a meal should be measured. If the blood glucose is equal to or greater than 10 mmol/1 (venous whole blood) or 11 mmol/1 (venous plasma or capillary whole blood) then the diagnosis is established.

If the blood value is greater than 7 mmol/1 but less than 10 mmol/1 then a modified GTT should be performed as above. It is important not to label a patient with the diagnosis of diabetes mellitus if he is not diabetic and until the diagnosis has been established on the basis of blood glucose values. The label may have important consequences with respect to life insurance, pension rights, driving and job prospects.

Impaired glucose tolerance is not diabetes and should not be labelled as such. However, it should not be ignored since it carries the risk of increased infant morbidity and mortality in pregnancy and an overall increase in cardiovascular morbidity and mortality. Simple preventative measures – such as weight loss, a high fibre diet, blood pressure control and blood lipid control should be instituted.

1.5 THE SYNDROME OF DIABETES MELLITUS

As indicated in section 1.1, diabetes mellitus is not a single disease entity but a group of diseases. Failure to recognize this fact has caused and still causes considerable confusion. The recognition that the syndrome of diabetes mellitus and its long-term complications can be caused by several aetiological processes has been an important step in the understanding of the disease.

Broadly speaking the nature of the diabetic syndrome produced is related to the degree of islet cell damage caused by the disease. It is also related to the degree of insulin resistance which the patient may have. For example, if a surgeon removes a pancreas the patient becomes immediately a totally insulin-dependent diabetic and requires insulin to be given to prevent hyperglycaemia, ketoacidosis and to prevent the development of coma and eventual death. On the other hand, the elderly obese patient may have only a relative lack of insulin and a high degree of insulin resistance. This would require treatment with diet alone with calorie restriction in order to lose weight and restore insulin sensitivity.

It is important at this stage to rid oneself of the dangerous concept of 'mild' diabetes. There is no such thing. This erroneous concept is usually based on the type of treatment the patient is receiving. The theoretically 'mild' diabetes of non-insulin dependent diabetics treated with diet alone when ignored can maim and kill. Most diabetologists will recall patients with 'mild' diabetes, confined to a wheelchair, blind, hemiplegic, and having had one or both legs amputated. By no stretch of the imagination can this be called 'mild'. By contrast some insulin-dependent diabetics live for many years with healthy bodies, free from long-term complications.

The classification of diabetes mellitus is as follows (WHO Expert Committee on Diabetes, 1980):

1. Insulin-dependent diabetes mellitus (IDDM).
2. Non-insulin dependent diabetes mellitus (NIDDM):
   (i) Non-obese.
   (ii) Obese.
3. Other types of diabetes mellitus related to:
   (i) Pancreatic disease/surgery
   (ii) Other endocrine syndromes, e.g. Cushing's syndrome.
   (iii) Iatrogenic disease (drugs and chemically induced).
   (iv) Certain genetic syndromes, e.g. MODY.
   (v) Miscellaneous causes.

Insulin dependence is defined as diabetes that requires insulin treatment from within 3 months of diagnosis and/or with episodes of ketoacidosis.

It is important to note that non-insulin dependent diabetes mellitus may be treated with insulin to obtain good glycaemic control.

The old term 'juvenile onset diabetes' is not synonymous with insulin-dependent diabetes mellitus since IDDM can occur at any age. However, it is more common in the younger age groups. Juvenile onset diabetes really refers to IDDM occurring in the young. Similarly, the term 'maturity onset diabetes' is not synonymous with non-insulin dependent diabetes mellitus since this syndrome may also occur in the young.

Type 1 diabetes mellitus is sometimes used when referring to

IDDM and type 2 diabetes mellitus to NIDDM. The terminology should be understood as it is used in much of the literature. However, it is probably better that the terms be discarded.

1.6 AETIOLOGY

IDDM occurring in the young is associated with certain inherited histocompatibility antigens (HLA systems) coupled with environmental attack from certain viruses, notably Coxsackie B4 and 5. Thus environmental factors acting on a susceptible individual appear to stimulate the production of autoimmune islet cell antibodies and complement fixing islet cell antibodies which eventually cause islet cell damage and insulin dependent diabetes mellitus. The genetic basis of IDDM is thus weak and related to the inheritance of histocompatibility antigens. On the other hand, genetic factors appear to be more important in non-insulin dependent diabetes mellitus. For example, if one identical twin develops non-insulin dependent diabetes mellitus, then it is almost certain that the other twin will develop NIDDM in the not too distant future. Again, there is an interaction between the environment on the one hand and a genetic susceptibility on the other. Obesity plays an important part in the genesis of non-insulin dependent diabetes mellitus in some patients.

Non-insulin dependent diabetes mellitus in the young, the so-called MODY syndrome (Maturity Onset Diabetes in the Young) is a dominantly inherited genetic disorder.

Enough has been said to indicate the complexity of the various disease processes that produce the syndrome of diabetes mellitus. Further treatment of this aspect of the subject is beyond the scope of this book.

1.7 SHORT-TERM EFFECTS OF HYPERGLYCAEMIA

Islet cell damage eventually leads to poor glucose homeostasis and hyperglycaemia. Depending on the severity of the hyperglycaemia the effects may be dramatic or subtle. As the blood glucose concentration increases it exceeds the renal threshold for the absorption of glucose and glycosuria results. At an early stage (sometimes many years) before symptoms occur, diabetes mellitus may be discovered after suspicion has been aroused because of glycosuria detected on routine urine testing when attending outpatients or for an insurance medical. Often hyperglycaemia with a little polyuria and polydipsia grumbles on for weeks, months or even years. Symptoms are often accompanied by weight loss. The osmotic effect of the glycosuria may eventually cause polyuria and relative dehydration. The latter gives rise to polydipsia. The excessive thirst is often the primary problem in the patient's mind. The polyuria is regarded as a consequence of the excessive drinking induced by the thirst.

If the dehydration is severe, hypovolaemia, hypotension, shock, and coma may develop (Chapter 5). This is more likely to be the case if insulin lack is so severe that the hepatic production of glucose and ketoacids is not inhibited. The patient then not only becomes dehydrated but also ketoacidotic and may develop diabetic ketoacidotic coma (DKA) (Chapter 5).

This natural history highlights the importance of asking routine questions in the history relating to appetite, weight and micturition. If you do not ask, you may not be told. It also indicates the importance of routine testing of the urine for glycosuria.

There is good laboratory experimental evidence to support the clinical impression that hyperglycaemic patients do have a diminished ability to respond to infection. There is also evidence to suggest that normoglycaemia restores the normal response. Unfortunately infection produces hyperglycaemia and the vicious circle of infection–hyperglycaemia–worsening infection is established.

The usual everyday infections are more severe and more frequent in diabetics. Tooth decay and gingivitis is often overlooked. Sinus infections are common and in elderly diabetics who are poorly controlled a particularly malignant type of mastoiditis may develop resulting in the death of the patient. For some reason this is rarely seen in the United Kingdom but has been reported more frequently in the United States. Infection of the skin, particularly by bacteria producing boils and furuncles, is a common mode of presentation in non-insulin dependent diabetics. Fungal infections, particularly between the toes, occur frequently in diabetics and are often missed. This is of great importance since a fungal infection may damage the skin barrier and allow the introduction of bacterial infection. In a foot under threat from neuropathy and vascular disease, the development of a fungal infection may lead to a rapidly spreading bacterial infection with loss of the foot (see Chapter 11, Diabetic

Foot Disease). It is essential to detect minor fungal and other infections of the foot and treat them vigorously.

Ulceration of the legs or feet, a failure to heal or slow healing should prompt further investigation of blood glucose levels.

Genitourinary tract infections may be asymptomatic. Any patient with symptoms or presenting with proteinuria should have a urine sample cultured and microscopically examined.

When treating infection normoglycaemia should be the aim. Normoglycaemia, particularly post operatively, reduces the risk of infection.

1.8 LONG-TERM EFFECTS OF HYPERGLYCAEMIA

With the introduction of effective methods of glucose control (insulin, 1921–22; sulphonylureas, 1945) the life span of the diabetic was increased. However, it soon became clear that with an increased life span the chance of developing what are now known as long-term complications increased. The long-term complications are responsible for the increased morbidity and mortality in diabetes. Diabetologists are now addressing the problem of defining the causes of long-term complications and determining ways of preventing or at least delaying their development. Clinically, emphasis has been laid on early detection and treatment of complications as they arise.

1.8.1 Aetiology

Hyperglycaemia appears to be associated with three main pathophysiological processes. The first involves damage of small vessels at the capilliary and arteriolar level. This is known as microvascular disease. The second involves larger vessels and produces early and advanced atherosclerotic changes. This is macrovascular disease. In addition to this disordered metabolism appears to be the main factor affecting the lens of the eye and nerves. These pathological processes rarely if ever act in isolation. Diabetic eye disease and diabetic renal disease are predominatly microvascular but may be complicated and made worse by macrovascular disease and hypertension. In addition diabetic renal disease may be complicated by infection producing pyelonephritis and occasionally papillary necrosis. Autonomic neuropathy affecting the bladder may also complicate diabetic renal disease. The heart is affected by microvascular disease and autonomic neuropathy but this is insignificant compared with the major impact of macrovascular disease (coronary artery disease). Nerve tissue damaged by the metabolic defect occurring in diabetes produces peripheral neuropathy but such nerves are also vulnerable to microvascular disease. However, the most florid example of multiple factors producing disease in the diabetic is diabetic foot disease. Here severe ischaemia may be produced by the localized or diffuse atherosclerosis of macrovascular disease. Microvascular disease may play a small part in devitalizing tissues. Autonomic neuropathy can produce significant shunting of blood away from the tissues of the foot. The presence of a peripheral neuropathy with altered sensation robs the patient of warning signs of trauma. If infection is added, the whole disastrous mix of pathological process proceeds apace with the risk of gangrene and subsequent amputation.

The most important aetiological factor in the development of long-term complications is hyperglycaemia. One large study of 4400 patients between 1947 and 1973 (Pirart, 1978) showed an increasing incidence of neuropathy, retinopathy and nephropathy with decreasing standards of glycaemic control. Time is also important. After 15–20 years duration of diabetes 80% of diabetics will have some evidence of diabetic retinopathy.

Glycaemia and time cannot be the only factors operating in the production of long-term complications. Most diabetologists look after patients who have had diabetes for 20 or 30 years and are free of overt complications. Other patients have had diabetes for a long time and have exhibited rather poor glycaemic control and yet do not have long-term complications. Even more dramatic are those patients who present (even acutely with insulin dependent diabetes) with a severe blinding retinopathy or the nephrotic syndrome due to diabetic nephropathy. Such patients are rare but they do indicate that there must be factors other than time and glycaemia affecting the development of long-term complications. The rate of development and severity of long-term complications of diabetes is very variable even in similarly controlled patients. The cause is almost certainly multifactorial. The common factor is hyperglycaemia acting on a possible genetic susceptibility in association with other hormonal abnormalities and environmental factors. Genetic susceptibility may be associated with immunogenetic factors. An increased incidence of complications has been reported in those patients having the histocompatibility antigens HLAB8, B15, and DR4. However, there is perhaps a stronger association with those patients exhibiting C4 B3 (the fourth component of complement) with an increased relative risk of 2.4. The presence of Gm (zagfmb) (the coding for IG heavy chain constant region) confers an increased relative risk of 4.1. The presence of both these factors increases the relative risk to 21 strongly suggesting that there is an immunogenetic component to microangiopathy.

Excessive growth hormone production has been reported in some patients with retinopathy compared with similarly controlled patients without retinopathy.

Smoking is an important example of an environmental factor having profound effects on macrovascular disease.

It is not the intention in this book to cover this subject in depth. For such a study the interested reader is referred to Keen and Jarret (1982). It is, however, intended to deal with those subjects of greater practical importance to the practising diabetologist and those members of the health care team looking after diabetics on a daily basis.

1.8.2 Classification

The manifestations of the complications of diabetes mellitus are as follows:

1. Microvascular disease:
   (i) Diabetic retinopathy (Chapter 7).
   (ii) Diabetic nephropathy (Chapter 8).
   (iii) Skin disorders.
   (iv) Increased bone fragility.
   (v) Diabetic cardiomyopathy.
2. Macrovascular disease (Chapter 9):
   (i) Peripheral vascular disease.
   (ii) Coronary artery disease.
   (iii) Cerebrovascular disease.
3. Metabolic disorders:
   (i) Diabetic neuropathy (Chapter 10).
   (ii) Cataracts (Chapter 7).
4. Reduced resistance to infection:
   (i) Gingivitis.
   (ii) Sinus infection.
   (iii) Infection of the skin (bacterial/fungal).

   (iv) Genitourinary tract infections.
5. Multifactorial problems:
   (i) Mononeuritis and mononeuritis multiplex (Chapter 10).
   (ii) Diabetic foot disease (Chapter 11).
6. Other – in pregnancy (Chapter 6):
   (i) Sub-fertility.
   (ii) Miscarriages.
   (iii) Stillbirth.
   (iv) Neonatal deaths.
   (v) Congenital defects.

Microvascular disease affects all tissues but principally the eye producing diabetic retinopathy (Chapter 7), and the kidney producing diabetic nephropathy (Chapter 8). Necrobiosis lipoidica diabeticorum is a disfiguring skin lesion for which there is unfortunately no specific treatment (Plate 1). Increased bone fragility may result from the microvascular disease. The increased bone resorption may make diabetics more prone to fractures. The significance of microvascular disease affecting the myocardium is in doubt and is overshadowed by the effects of macrovascular disease.

Macrovascular disease produces coronary artery disease, cerebrovascular disease and peripheral vascular disease. Ischaemia of the legs and feet is often associated with neuropathy and infection (Chapter 11).

Vascular disease affecting the vasanervorum produces mononeuritis and mononeuritis multiplex. However, disorders of metabolism associated with hyperglycaemia cause abnormal nerve function and result in peripheral neuropathy. Similar metabolic abnormalities affect the autonomic nerves resulting in autonomic neuropathy (Chapter 10). This metabolic abnormality is probably related to disorder d-polyol metabolism in nerve tissue with the accumulation of sorbitol. A similar mechanism may be responsible for the development of cataract (Chapter 7).

From the practical point of view it is clear that although we are not as yet able to change genetic susceptibility, we can attempt to produce normal or near-normal glycaemia and persuade patients to stop smoking.

1.9 THE SIZE OF THE PROBLEM

The prevalance of diabetes mellitus is different in different ethnic populations and in each age group within the population. In a predominantly white (Caucasian) population having the age/sex structure of the United Kingdom, 1.01% of the population will have diabetes. However, 3.5% of those over the age of 65 years will have diabetes and more than 50% of all diabetics will be over the age of 65 years. With an ageing population this problem of numbers is likely to become an important factor for consideration in the provision of health care (Gatling *et al.*, 1985).

A doctor engaged in primary health care looking after a population of say 2500 patients will have approximately 20 – 25 patients with diabetes mellitus under his care. A district general hospital caring for a population of 250 000 patients will have in excess of 2500 patients potentially attending the diabetic clinic. This large number of patients which requires constant monitoring and follow-up presents logistical problems of health care provision and this will be discussed later. (Chaper 13).

1.10 MORBIDITY

The overall disability rates in diabetics are 2–3 times higher than in non-diabetics.

In the USA 25% of all patients reaching end-stage renal failure requiring dialysis or transplantation are diabetics.

Diabetes is the single most common cause of blindness in the UK.

Gangrene of the lower limbs requiring amputation is 20 – 30 times more common in diabetics than in non-diabetics.

1.11 MORTALITY

The overall life expectancy of a patient developing diabetes in childhood is only 50% of that expected by a non-diabetic control. Even those developing diabetes in later life lose 30% of their expected life span.

The mortality associated with coronary thrombosis is twice that of non-diabetic controls.

Macrovascular disease is responsible for a large proportion of the increased mortality associated with diabetes particularly in non-insulin dependent diabetes. However, renal failure accounts for a large proportion of the increased mortality amongst those developing diabetes under the age of 20.

1.12 CONCLUSION

The syndrome of diabetes mellitus is common. Its cost is high both in economic terms and in terms of mortality and morbidity. It requires thorough and systematic care. To provide this only an organized team approach will be effective if large numbers of patients are to be coped with. It is the aim of this book to outline such an approach. Only by the effective organization of the health care service will the diabetic gain the health care he so desperately needs.

REFERENCES

Gatling, W., Houston, A.C., and Hill, R.D. (1985) The prevalence of diabetes mellitus in a typical English community. *Journal of the Royal College of Physicians of London*, **19**, 248.

Keen, H. and Jarrett, R. J. (eds) (1982) *Complications of Diabetes*, 2nd edn. Edward Arnold, London.

Pirart, J. (1978) Diabetes mellitus and its degenerative complications : A prospective study of 4400 patients observed between 1947 and 1973. *Diabetes Care*, **1**, 168–188, 252–63.

WHO Expert Committee on Diabetes Mellitus (1980) *2nd Report*, Technical Report Series 646. WHO, Geneva.

· Two ·

Making the diagnosis and initiating treatment

2.1 WHO SHOULD BE SCREENED FOR GLYCOSURIA?

Modern computer systems are able to run self-diagnostic programmes to detect faults. Evolution has not yet equipped the human race with such a programme. In the event we can only suspect the possibility of a disorder and then run the appropriate tests to confirm or refute the suspicion. However, patients may have hyperglycaemia for many years without symptoms and present with a blinding retinopathy, neuropathy, or macrovascular disease. How is this to be prevented?

The aim of screening is to discover the presence of a disorder in its early stages with the hope that early treatment will prevent or lessen damage to the individual. Perhaps the perfect screening test in this context would be that every individual should have a blood glucose measured 2 hours after a meal rich in carbohydrate as an annual event. Clearly this is not a practical proposition in the real world. A urine test for glucose collected after a meal rich in carbohydrate might be a suitable screening substitute. In this test the patient is advised to empty the bladder, have a meal rich in carbohydrate, and 2 hours later empty the bladder and this specimen is then tested for glucose. If such a screening test were to be performed on a large population only 1–2 patients per 100 tested would reveal glycosuria and eventually have the diagnosis of diabetes confirmed. At least half of these patients would already be known to be diabetic. The cost of such a screening test would be extremely high in relation to the benefit obtained and it is unlikely that this could be considered as a practical possibility. Who then should be tested for glycosuria? The following should have a urine test for glucose:

1. Symptoms suggesting an osmotic diuresis – polydipsia, polyuria, nocturia, incontinence.

2. Symptoms suggesting a change in plasma osmolarity – changes in visual acuity, thirst.
3. Changes in weight – weight loss or obesity.
4. Recurrent infections, particularly of the skin – cellulitis with or without ulceration, boils, balanitis, pruritus vulvac and intertrigo.
5. Neuropathic symptoms – pain, numbness and paraesthesia affecting legs and feet.
6. Peripheral vascular disease – intermittent claudication, ischaemic skin, ulceration and gangrene.
7. Coronary artery disease – angina pectoris and myocardial infarction.
8. Transient ischaemic attacks (TIA) and stroke.
9. Family history of diabetes in first-degree relatives, particularly in the event of unexplained fetal loss.
10. All females with a history of giving birth to large babies (i.e. birth weight greater than 4 kg).
11. Unexplained fetal loss.
12. Unexplained symptoms.
13. Insurance medical examinations.
14. Routine medical examinations.
15. ? Practice screening programmes.

Here it is important to stress the necessity for good history taking. This is an art learnt at medical school and often forgotten after qualifying. If you do not ask the right questions then you will not get relevant answers. Two minutes spent asking the patient about appetite, weight, and micturition often reveals unexpected symptoms about which the patient did not bother to complain. Diabetes mellitus is a common disease. The diagnosis will only be made by maintaining a high index of suspicion.

2.2 ACTION TO BE TAKEN ON FINDING GLYCOSURIA

If glycosuria is discovered the diagnosis of diabetes mellitus must be confirmed to WHO criteria (see sections 1.3 and 1.4).

Figure 2.1 shows the decision-making pathway to be taken on finding glycosuria. The often omitted essential step is the test for ketonuria. The presence of ketones must be interpreted in the light of

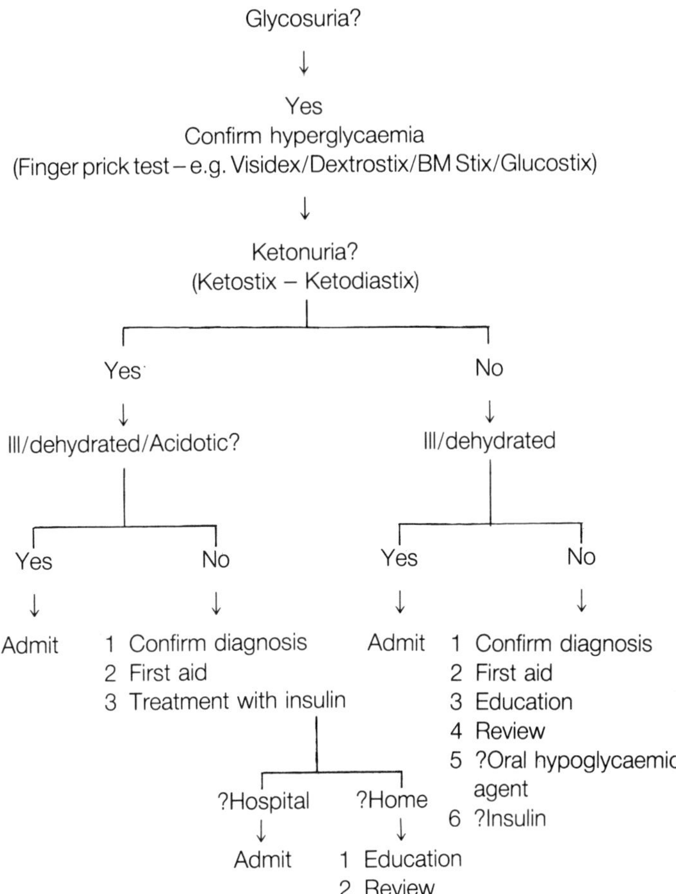

Figure 2.1 Action to be taken on finding glycosuria.

clinical findings. Ketonuria can occur in the obese on a very low carbohydrate diet. In the child or in the thin adult when it is often associated with weight loss, it may indicate the early stages of life-threatening diabetic ketoacidosis.

CAUTION: In children extreme caution should be exercised. On finding glycosuria the advice of a local paediatric department or diabetic specialist (if he looks after the children in the area) should be sought. The rapidity with which children may become severely ill cannot be overemphasized. An early diagnosis may mean that a child can be treated at home with the help of a diabetic specialist nurse. The child is then saved from the trauma of admission to hospital, intravenous therapy and all that this entails. Similar caution should be exercised in the thin adult with glycosuria, ketonuria and weight loss.

The time course of the decision-making pathway varies from a few hours in the case of diabetic ketoacidosis, to a few days where the diagnosis is in doubt. However, once the diagnosis is established and the urgency of the situation determined, then treatment must begin with first aid.

2.3 FIRST AID

First aid is that advice and help given to the patient at diagnosis. It may be divided into three parts:

1. Reassurance.
2. Dietary advice.
3. Self-monitoring.

2.3.1 Reassurance

On learning the diagnosis a newly diagnosed diabetic is often shocked and frightened. He is frightened by the unknown or by the partially known with its hints of 'blindness', 'gangrene', and 'early death'. The reaction is often that of disbelief and rejection of the diagnosis. This reaction may soon be followed by resentment and rebellion with an attitude of non-co-operation and non-compliance. After a variable period the patient may come to terms with the situation and accept the diagnosis. With acceptance comes co-operation, compliance, and general peace of mind.

The time course of these stages varies from individual to individual and according to the age of patient and the type of diabetes. In my experience the middle aged and elderly more readily accept the diagnosis and rapidly pass through the various stages to acceptance and co-operation. Most of these patients will be non-insulin dependent diabetics. As one might expect, the young insulin dependent diabetic is upset most severely. Adolescence is a difficult time for all and to have a life-long sentence of diabetes mellitus in addition may be the straw that breaks the emotional camel's back. It is not surprising, therefore, that these patients require the most careful handling if a prolonged period of resentment and rebellion is to be avoided.

Whether the patient is young or old, insulin dependent or non-insulin dependent, this aspect of diabetic care must not be omitted. The diabetic with ketoacidosis and dehydration who at the outset requires admission to hospital is often overwhelmed by events with the associated i.v. infusions, injections of insulin, and all the paraphernalia of intensive care. Initially they are relieved and indeed thankful to be still alive. However, soon the full realization of the situation dawns. It is often forgotten that it is at this point, when the drama is over, that the patient needs most psychological support.

In the non-insulin dependent diabetic the drama may not be there but nevertheless patients still have fears and must be reassured. Whether the diagnosis is made in primary health care by the family doctor, or in secondary health care by the hospital doctor, the medical attitude should be one of quiet, gentle sympathetic reassurance coupled with simple and brief explanation. Allow the patient to ask quesions. Do not give complicated explanations. Little will be remembered at this stage. Give the diabetic time to consider the situation and return later with more questions. The properly managed diabetic will later be given the opportunity to attend a diabetic education session and gain more detailed knowledge.

Initially the explanation should be confined to the following points:

1. Diabetes is a disorder in which there is too much sugar (glucose) in the blood.
2. This sugar (glucose) can be found in the urine by a suitable simple test.
3. Diabetes is a treatable condition although treatment may last for life.
4. Long-term problems are not inevitable.
5. The diabetic can lead a full, and useful and near-normal life (NB International sportsmen and women, transatlantic yachtsmen, famous actors and actresses, etc.).

The emphasis should be on the positive aspects of advice rather than the negative ones. Emphasize the 'do's' rather than the 'don'ts'.

Figure 2.2 Community care service for diabetics in the Poole area. Letter to patient.

Dear patient,

If your diabetes is newly diagnosed you will no doubt be anxious about the future. Let us reassure you right away that with proper care and treatment you will be able to live a full and normal life. You may feel better than your non-diabetic friends! Even if you have had diabetes for some time you may be apprehensive about what sort of service we will provide. You will be pleased to hear that you are in a district which makes a special effort to care for those with diabetes.

There is a team* of workers helping **you** to look after **yourself** and manage **your** diabetes. **REMEMBER THAT THE MOST IMPORTANT PERSON IN THE HEALTH CARE TEAM LOOKING AFTER THE DIABETIC IS YOU.**

Your first introduction to the service has already taken place when you consulted your own family doctor. Your next contact with the service will be at the Diabetic Education Session. You should attend promptly at the time you have been given, and you must expect to be there two or three hours. There you will be given an introduction to diabetes, advice on diet, information about the Diabetic Service, and taught many other things relating to diabetes. The Education Session is run by the **Diabetic Liaison Sister** and the **Dietitian.** The session is informal and friendly and you will be given plenty of time to ask questions. You will not need to see a doctor on this occasion unless there is some urgent need. This will be arranged by the Diabetic Liaison Sister. During this Education Session you will be given an appointment for the Diabetic Clinic. Please do not leave the session without detting this appointment.

Before coming to the Diabetic Education Session may we offer this simple advice on your diet:

- Avoid all sweetened drinks, jams, marmalade and honey. **Low calorie or sugar free drinks, and sugar free preserves may be used.**
- Do not eat sugary puddings or deserts, tinned fruit in syrup, tinned milk puddings, or jellies. **Instead, eat fresh or stewed fruit using a sugar free sweetener if necessary, or fruit tinned without sugar.**
- Avoid all sweet biscuits, cakes, sweets, and chocolates. **If you are hungry between meals eat fruit.**
- Do not eat low fibre starchy foods such as low fibre white bread, flour, crisp breads, biscuits, breakfast cereals, white pasta, or rice. **Instead, have fibre rich foods such as wholemeal bread and flour, high fibre crisp breads, biscuits and breakfast cereals, wholemeal pasta and brown rice, jacket potatoes and vegetables such as peas and beans.**

Your meals can be planned in your normal way – providing you have cut out

* Nurses, dietitians, chiropodists, laboratory workers, pharmacists, secretaries, and doctors, together with other workers both in the community and in the hospital.

the sugar and refined foods, as this will start to bring your diabetes under control.

If you are also overweight, you should reduce the amount of fat you eat by using less butter, margarine, oil, lard, dripping and cheese.

This is stop-gap advice for you to follow until you see the dietitian who will plan a personal diet with you.

Please complete this questionnaire and bring it with you when you come to the Diabetic Education Session. It will help our Medical Records Department.

IDENTITY

Mr/Mrs/Miss/Ms.

Surname..

1st Forename..

2nd Forename ....

NHS Number ....
(from your NHS card or your doctor's receptionist)

Address..

....

....

Postcode...

Telephone number (Home) ....

(Work)..

Date of Birth ....

Next of Kin

Name ....

Address..

....

....

Post Code ....

Telephone number...............................

Relationship...

General Practitioner

Name ....

Address..

....

....

Post Code ....

REMEMBER

Look forward to a healthier life!
Attend the next Diabetic Education Session as instructed.
Test your urine once daily or as instructed by your doctor.
Take the simple advice given above.

We look forward to meeting you.

Yours sincerely

2.3.2 Dietary advice

Initial dietary advice must be simple and should be confined to advice on abstaining from those foods containing mono and disaccharides. It is surprising how many patients improve dramatically and often become asymptomatic (though not necessarily well controlled) with simple dietary advice alone.

Figure 2.2 illustrates a letter given by family doctors to all patients at diagnosis or on referral. This gives simple dietary advice, reassurance, and an introduction to the diabetic education session.

2.3.3 Self-monitoring

It is important at the outset to introduce the patient to the concept that 'the most important person in the Health Care Team looking after the diabetic is the diabetic'. This should be coupled with the idea of 'self-monitoring'. Initially this should be by urine testing for glucose (Diastix (Ames), Diabur-Test 500 (MCP)).

Foster the attitude:

I test myself.
I review the results.
I take action.

Initially the 'action' may be limited to reporting the results to the doctor since the patient's own knowledge will be limited. However, in the next stage in the management of the diabetic, that of education, the aim is to make the diabetic self-reliant and self-sufficient:

> 'You must manage your own diabetic state – we will provide all the help we can – if you do not look after yourself no one else will.'

· Three ·

Educating the diabetic

3.1 INTRODUCTION

One of the important advances in diabetic care has been the recognition that the most important person in the Health Care Team looking after the diabetic is the diabetic. That this change was necessary is clear from reviews of the standard of glycaemic control achieved by conventional methods. In children only 1.5% achieved haemoglobin Al concentrations within the normal range. (Mann and Johnson, 1982) and only 11–13% of adults approached within three standard deviations of the normal (Tattersall and McCulloch, 1984). This has involved a change in the attitude of the diabetologist from that of authoritarian to that of adviser. It has required the devolution of responsibility from the doctor to the patient. Our purpose is not to force patients into taking a particular course of action but only to advise what, in the light of our knowledge and experience, we think is the best course for the patient's well being. Thus the patient must not only take advantage of our knowledge and skills but also our experience and judgement. Therefore there must be an element of trust between doctor and patient. Paternalism is not dead!

> 'Communication is of crucial importance in medicine. Partly to inform, explain, and advise, and partly – especially when the patient is frightened, ill, weak or otherwise vulnerable – to raise morale, give confidence, encourage, and protect. Whether or not we call this 'paternalism', the fact is that to try to abolish it would be a sure way to add greatly to the sum of total human suffering.'
>
> (Brewin, 1985)

Examination of patients' knowledge about their diabetes has revealed major deficiencies (Etzwiler and Sines, 1962; Beaser, 1956; Miller *et al.*, 1978). If the patient is to accept the responsibility for his or her own health care rather than to rely totally on others, then a new responsibility falls upon the Health Care Team. This must be to provide the educational facilities matched to the patient's own abilities and capacity to learn. Although patient education does not necessarily produce behavioural change, education can improve glycaemic control as indicated by haemoglobin A1 values (McCulloch *et al.*, 1983). In addition, if coupled with a 24 hour service staffed by diabetic nurse specialists, dramatic reductions in admission rates, diabetic ketoacidosis and amputation rates can be achieved (Miller and Goldstein, 1972). At this point it is worth while setting out clearly the aims of educating the diabetic. These are to

1. Encourage the patient to accept the responsibility for his or her own health care.
2. Encourage the patient to acquire the necessary information.
3. Encourage the patient to alter his or her behaviour in the light of the acquired information.

The acquisition of knowledge does not necessarily imply a change in behaviour. The smoker who is aware of the dangers of smoking continues to smoke!

If we are to achieve these aims then we must first consider the 'learning process'.

3.2 THE LEARNING PROCESS

The learning process may be summarized as follows:

1. Aims – the acquisition of information and to achieve a change in behaviour.
2. Steps:
   (i) Motivation.
   (ii) Attention.
   (iii) Acquisition of data.
   (iv) Retention.
   (v) Recall.
   (vi) Applications.
   (vii) Performance – action.
   (viii) Behavioural change.

Motivation is the first and vital step on the road to self-sufficiency. Shortly after diagnosis the patient will come into contact with doctors, nurses, dietitians, chiropodists, and many others (including other diabetics). The personalities and apparent attitudes expressed by these contacts will have a profound effect on the attitude of the patient. It is essential for all these workers to speak with one voice and that there should be no conflict in attitudes, views, or information. There must be understanding, sympathy and enthusiasm, but above all there must be optimism and a firm belief in an improved standard of health and well being. The interest of the patient should be stimulated to achieve a more healthy and happy life.

Once the patient's interest has been aroused and he has been motivated to improve his own standard of health care then it is important to present educational material to the patient in such a way that his attention is gained and maintained.

Information is presented to the patient in many different ways. If we hope to stimulate the patient to acquire knowledge, there is little point in just handing out a printed sheet of information in the hope that the educational process will proceed automatically. However, the printed word must not be discarded. It should be used as an adjunct to other teaching aids shown in (2)–(7) below:

1. The printed word.
2. Face to face group teaching (large/small) – i.e. lecture/discussion.
3. Video presentations (group large/small).
4. Slide – tape presentations.
5. Small group practical teaching sessions.
6. Face to face – one to one tutorials.
7. Interactive computer teaching programes with assessment and prescriptive feedback.

It must be remembered that most patients will have little or no biological background knowledge. The information presented in the education sessions therefore represents a vast amount of new data to be acquired. The acquisition of data is of little use if it is not retained. In the conventional face-to-face group teaching method, i.e. the formal lecture, retention is only about 5% and yet this is the most widely used method of teaching! At the other end of the scale the use of an interactive computer program enables the patient to move forward step by step with the computer testing the acquisition of data before allowing the patient to move on to the next step. If the patient can read and understand simple English, and can understand and act on simple instructions, the method is suitable for the young and selected patients of an older age group. The program teaches, asks relevant questions to assess reaction and understanding, and the patient answers through the simplified keyboard. This has keys corresponding to digits 0–9, Yes, No, and Do Not Know. The patient cannot move on to the next step of the program until he understands the preceding stage. The learning is therefore paced to coincide with the individual's capacity to learn.

After initial presentations it is important that revision should be a continuous process in order to establish long-term memory and adequate recall of information.

It is important to have some means of evaluating the amount of information acquired by the patient and how much of this information is retained. Simple questionnaires and optical mark readers may be used to give a numerical assessment of the patient's knowledge. Simple computer programs are also available to provide an assessment of the patient's knowledge to indicate weak areas and to allow the educator to concentrate on those areas that require revision. Programs are even available which will provide 'prescriptive feedback'. At the end of a computer teaching session there is an assessment session which then provides a printout for the patient giving details of answers which were incorrect and giving the correct answer. By repeating the process the patient acquires information, is assessed, and his progress followed.

When educating the diabetic a combination of teaching methods should be used. These will vary according to the individual's requirements. The education process must be ongoing and give the patient the opportunity to discuss all aspects of diabetes in order to assess how much information he or she has retained and that recall of this information is possible.

Assessing the patient's ability to apply acquired knowledge is more difficult. However, the overall assessment of the standard of control achieved by the diabetic and the maintenance of ideal body weight will indicate how well the diabetic is applying his knowledge, taking action with respect to this knowledge, and even perhaps changing a previously established behavioural pattern.

3.3 THE SYLLABUS

Individual physicians will have their own ideas as to what should be taught in the diabetic education session. The ability of the patient to cope with the educational programme will depend on intelligence, educational, social and racial background, and age.

An outline of a syllabus (used by the Community Care Service for

Diabetics in the Poole Area, 1986) is as follows:

1. What is diabetes mellitus?
2. Diet and diabetes. Eating for a healthy life.
3. Self-monitoring – (i) Urine testing.
4. Foot care.
5. Eye care.
6. What do we mean by good diabetic control?
7. Co-operation and the co-operation book.
8. Life with diabetes (exercise, smoking, illness and driving).
9. On transfer to GP care. Your reminder.
10. Treatment with insulin.
11. Self-monitoring – (ii) home blood glucose monitoring.
12. Advanced 'postgraduate' sessions for insulin taking diabetics.

The subjects covered by (1)–(8) are for all diabetics; (9) covers important information for patients transferred to family doctor (GP) care for routine diabetic follow-up. The subject matter of (10) is for patients who are treated with insulin and that of (11) for selected insulin treated diabetics who wish to monitor their own blood glucose at home. The advanced postgraduate sessions are for young insulin taking diabetics. On the whole, this acts as a revision course and a problem-solving session.

3.3.1 What is diabetes mellitus?

This section is basically introductory. Group teaching is used catering for approximately eight or nine patients with a similar number of relatives. There is a short introductory talk by a specialist nursing sister followed by a slide/tape (talk-over) presentation. There then follows a discussion led by the clinical nurse specialist (Diabetic Liaison Sister)

3.3.2 Diet and diabetes. Eating for a healthy life

The initial part of this session is by group teaching. This caters for approximately nine patients with an equal number of relatives. There is an initial introductory talk in which it is stressed that patients are not being asked to go on a diet but to change their way of life and to eat 'healthily'. In this respect it is suggested that the dietary advice offered is for the whole family and not just for the patient.

The introductory talk is followed by a slide presentation. There is then a discussion led by the dietitian. Following the introductory session individual dietary histories are taken by dietitians and personal dietary advice given. This is on a one-to-one basis with a relative sitting in and taking part. This is usually essential where men are concerned since it is the wife who more often than not prepares the food. Follow-up dietary appointments are arranged by the dietitian who monitors the patient's weight and bears in mind the standard of control being achieved and the presence or absence of hyperlipidaemia.

3.3.3 Self-monitoring – (i) urine testing

Here small group (two or three) teaching is used for the initial introductory talk and practical demonstration. There follows individual tuition. Patients are advised on the frequency of testing and the charting of results. The concept of the most important person in the Health Care Team looking after the diabetic is the diabetic is stressed.

3.3.4 Foot care

Here large group teaching is used (eight or nine patients with an equal number of relatives). An introductory talk is given by a chiropodist and a slide/tape (talk-over) presentation is available. A free discussion follows led by the chiropodist. Individual chiropody appointments with examination, discussion, and further education are arranged by the chiropodist.

3.3.5 Eye care

The importance of not having a new pair of spectacles prescribed until the diabetes is controlled is emphasized. This subject is initially touched upon in the introductory talk on diabetes but is detailed in the one to one discussion during the consultation with the doctor. The doctor also introduces the danger of diabetic eye disease and stresses the importance of good diabetic (glycaemic) control and annual eye examinations.

3.3.6 What do we mean by diabetic control?

This subject is introduced in the introductory talk (What is Diabetes?). It is reintroduced in the dietary discussions. The subject is again discussed on a one-to-one basis with the doctor. The concept of a normal blood glucose range is introduced as is the use of the haemoglobin A1 as a measure of long-term control. The relationship between blood glucose levels and urine test is discussed. Home monitoring of urine or blood is discussed in relation to the individual patient. 'Normal' values are given and realistic goals are set for the patient to achieve. Similarly target weights are set for the patient.

3.3.7 Co-operation and the co-operation book

In group teaching sessions (specialist diabetic sister) and in one-to-one face-to-face discussions with the doctor, the importance of the individual in managing his or her own diabetes is stressed. The idea of a team or co-operative effort between the patient, primary health care, and secondary health care is introduced and explained. The Co-operation Book as a means of furthering this end and as a means of communication is introduced. The book is discussed page by page. Each patient is given a book with his or her own personal details and clinical record.

3.3.8 Life with diabetes

The subjects of smoking, exercise, and driving are discussed in relation to diabetes. The effects of intercurrent illness on diabetic control are explained. Advice on what to do during intercurrent illness is given.

These topics are all covered in the Co-operation Book which is reintroduced and revised.

3.3.9 On transfer to GP care

This explains to patients what is expected of a patient and what is expected of a family doctor when a patient is transferred for routine follow up to the general practitioner's (GP) care. Again the importance of the individual's responsibility for his or her own health care is stressed – 'If you do not look after yourself, no one else will'. The importance of adhering to dietary advice is stressed. An open invitation is given to contact the dietitian should any problems arise. A minimum twice yearly follow-up by the family doctor is advised. Patients are requested to obtain a 2 hour interval blood sugar and HbA1 2 weeks before attending the family doctor and are asked to ensure that the information is recorded in the Co-operation Book in order that they may see how well controlled they are. The relevance of home monitoring is similarly stressed and patients are asked to present their results to their family doctor. The importance of an annual eye examination, regular foot care, and blood pressure

Table 3.1 Transferred to GP Care. Your reminder. (Booklet, the Community Service for Diabetics in the Poole Area.)

Page 2 Diet: Continue with your diet. If you need help you should make an appointment to see the dietitian.	*Page 3* Blood tests: These should be done at least twice a year. Two weeks before your appointment, 2 hours after you start a main meal.
Page 4 **U**rine indicates standards of control. **R**eplace cap on Diastix bottle. **I**nstructions must be followed. **N**egative tests are the aim. **E**ven when negative do not stop.	*Page 5* **T**est once a day. **E**nter results on the chart. **S**how results to your doctor. **T**est at a different time.
Page 6 Eyes: You should have your eyes examined every year by an ophthalmic optician, an ophthalmic medical practitioner or an eye specialist.	*Page 7* Feet: Follow the advice in your co-operation book. Report all sore or discoloured areas to your doctor.
Page 8 Blood pressure. At least once every year you should have your blood pressure measured.	

measurement is reiterated. The booklet (as shown in *Table 3.1*) is used during this teaching period (given by the doctor transferring the patient to the family doctor's care), and the advice given is reinforced before the patient leaves the clinic by a slide/tape (talk-over) programme.

3.3.10 Treatment with insulin

This teaching programme is of necessity extensive. It is carried out either on the ward for patients admitted for conversion to insulin, or in the home by the clinical nurse specialist (Diabetic Liaison Sister). The subjects covered are as follows:

1. Why insulin is necessary.
2. Where insulin comes from.
3. Insulin storage.
4. The insulin syringe, its care, measuring the dose.
5. Drawing up insulin into the syringe.
6. Insulin mixing techniques.
7. Injection techniques, injection sites.
8. Hypoglycaemia, glucagon.
9. Illness.
10. Driving.

Teaching is done on a one to one basis, using videos and computer programmes and practical demonstrations.

With increasing competence and confidence, the patient is taught how to adjust the insulin dose.

3.3.11 Self-monitoring – (ii) Home blood glucose monitoring

Teaching is done on a one-to-one basis. The subjects covered are:

1. Finger-pricking techniques.
2. Getting an adequate quantity of blood on to the test strip.
3. The use of various meters.
4. The charting of results.

Firms supplying meters to the district provide teaching sessions on the use, maintenance, and standardization of instruments. They provide back-up cover and maintenance. Two firms are used in the district on the basis that competition is healthy. The firm providing the best service gets the most clients!

3.3.12 Advanced 'postgraduate' session for insulin taking diabetics

This postgraduate course is for insulin dependent diabetics. It is basically a refresher course covering most aspects of diabetes discussed in the previous sections. There is an emphasis on those areas particularly applicable to the insulin taking diabetic and there is a great deal of time for discussion. Diabetes and its relation to work, marriage, preconception control, pregnancy, and children is discussed. The session is designed to define and solve any problems for the individual.

3.4 METHODS OF PRESENTATION

The educator must be motivated, enthusiastic, knowledgeable and sympathetic. In order to cover the above syllabus it is essential to have two or three main education sessions for all diabetics. There will be two or three individual dietary consultations and at least one chiropody consultation. Other aspects of education such as treatment with insulin require special arrangements. Home blood glucose monitoring and the advanced postgraduate courses require special arrangements for groups of patients. The remainder of the education takes place during routine consultations with doctors and other members of the Health Care Team. It is therefore important that the team speaks with one voice and that no confusing information be given to the patient.

There are now available numerous audio-visual educational aids:

1. The printed word.
2. Acetates for overhead projection.
3. Slides.
4. Slide/tape programmes.
5. Audio cassettes.
6. Video cassettes.
7. Interactive computer teaching programs.

Some of those currently in use in 1986 are listed in section 3.6.

3.5 CONCLUSIONS

All diabetics, whether newly diagnosed or known diabetics new to the area, must attend the education session. We have found that new diabetics appreciate the programme and that known diabetics need re-educating. Known diabetics, particularly those of some years standing and usually thinking that they 'know it all', are usually in great need of re-education. There is often an initial resistance but after the programme there is almost universal praise and appreciation. The initial resistance can usually be overcome by explaining that even a diabetologist needs constant update and revision since our knowledge about diabetes is continually advancing.

3.6 EDUCATING THE DIABETIC – AUDIO-VISUAL AIDS

3.6.1 What is diabetes?

1. Produced by the British Diabetic Association, 10 Queen Anne Street, London W1M 0BD.
   Introduction to Diabetes – a leaflet.
   Introduction to Diabetes – a tape/slide programme.
   Living with Diabetes by Dr Arnold Bloom.
   Diabetes Handbook. (i) Non-insulin dependent diabetes; (ii) Insulin dependent diabetes, by Dr John L. Day.
2. *Talking about Diabetes, Module 1* – What is Diabetes? Produced by BCL, Bell Lane, E. Sussex BN7 1LG, UK. Each module consists of acetates for overhead projection, a flip chart, a video, and a patient work book. It also contains a teacher's guide and slides are available on request. This is the first of a 14 module programme.

3.6.2 Diet and diabetes

1. 2 × 2 colour slides suitable for illustrating talks by dietitians are available from the British Diabetic Association, 10 Queen Anne Street, London W1M 0BD.
2. *A Guide for Diabetics*, a simple coloured visual aid produced by the Diabetic Department, Poole General Hospital, and the East Dorset Health Education Committee.
3. The dietary section in the Community Care Service Co-

operation Book (see Chapter 4).

4. The Poole General Hospital diet book available from the Dietetics Department, Poole General Hospital (see Chapter 4).
5. Video *Sugar Mountain Blues*, suitable for the teenager produced by and available from Nordisk, Highview House, Tattenham Crescent, Epsom, Surrey.
6. *Food Models* (reproductions) available from Replica Foods Limited, 73 Buckingham Avenue, Slough, Bucks, UK.
7. Cookery books:
   (i) *Simple Home Baking.*
   (ii) *Simple Home Cooking.*
   (iii) *Better Cooking for Diabetics.*
   (iv) *Cooking the New Diabetic Way.*

   All available from the British Diabetic Association, 10 Queen Anne Street, London W1M 0BD.

   Carbohydrate Count Down available from the British Diabetic Association, 10 Queen Anne Street, London W1M 0BD

   Carbohydrate Count Down Game available from the British Diabetic Association, 10 Queen Anne Street, London W1M 0BD.

   The Diabetics Diet Book, by Jim Mann and the Oxford Dietetic Group, published by Martin Dunitz in their positive Health Guide Series, available from book shops. This is an excellent book and should be basic reading for all. (Not only diabetics but for all those teaching diabetics.)
8. Computer Program

   The Diabetics' Diet Program. This is available from Martin Dunitz Ltd. This programme is a complex interactive computer dietary program which will not be suitable for all patients.

3.6.3 Self-monitoring – (i) Urine testing

The information contained in the urine testing strip bottles is sufficient to remind the patient of what has been taught in a practical session. There is no real substitute for one-to-one practical teaching.

3.6.4 Foot care

A section in the co-operation book advises and reminds patients of the importance of foot care.

Foot Care for Diabetics – slide/tape produced by Poole General

Hospital.

Various videos produced by the British Diabetic Association, 10 Queen Anne Street, London W1M 0BD, and as part of the modular series produced by BCL, Lewes, Bell Lane, E. Sussex BN7 1LG, UK.

3.6.5 Co-operation and Co-operation Record Book

The *Community Care Co-operation Book* is available from Hoechst Pharmaceuticals, Meducation Division, Salisbury Road, Hounslow, Middlesex, TW4 6GH and is free of charge.

3.6.6 Life with diabetes

The British Diabetic Association, 10 Queen Anne Street, London W1M 0B1).

Publications of the American Diabetes Association, 2 Park Avenue, New York, NY 10016, USA:

1. *Diabetes Care* reprints:
   (i) Principles of nutrition and dietary recommendations for individuals with diabetes mellitus : Special Report.
   (ii) Fructose, xylitol and sorbitol.
   (iii) Fast food restaurants.
   (iv) Office guide to diagnosis and classification of diabetes mellitus and other categories of glucose intolerance.
   (v) Indications for use of continuous insulin delivery systems and self-measurement of blood glucose.
   (vi) Third-party reimbursement for outpatient education and nutrition counselling.
   (vii) Glycaemic effects of carbohydrates.
2. Booklet: *A Guide for Professionals : The Effective Application of Exchange Lists for Meal Planning.*
3. Pamphlet: *A Word to . . . Pharmacists.*
4. Books:
   Curriculum for Youth Education.
   Diabetes Mellitus, 5th edn.
   The Physician's Guide to Type II Diabetes (NIDDM).

The Ames Educational Series (Ames Corporation, Miles Laboratories, PO Box 37, Stoke Court, Stoke Poges, Slough, SL2 4LY, UK):

1. *An Introduction to Diabetes.*

2. *An Introduction to Diet.*
3. *An Introduction to the Management of Children with Diabetes in Hospital.*
4. *Rupert and His Friends – A Guide for the Young Diabetic.*
5. *Rupert Teaches Dextrostix – A Guide for the Young Diabetic.*
6. *Self Urine Testing for Glucose and Ketones.*
7. *Self Blood Glucose Monitoring.*
8. *Good Health and Diabetes.*
9. *Non Insulin Dependent Diabetes.*
10. *Good Health and Insulin Dependent Diabetes.*

3.6.7 Transferred to GP care

This booklet may be obtained from (Servier Laboratories Ltd.) (For address see Section 3.6.11.)

3.6.8 Treatment with insulin

See various British Diabetic Association publications, 10 Queen Anne Street, London W1M 0BD. Various modules from the 14 module BCL series of teaching aids, including acetates, flip charts, video, patient workbook, and teacher's guide. Slides are also available on request. BCL, Bell Lane, Lewes, E. Sussex BN7 1LG, UK.

Adjustment of insulin dosage slide rule designed by Sister P. Hindley, Department of Diabetes, Poole General Hospital, and available from the Ames Corporation, Miles Laboratories Ltd. Ames Division, PO Box 37, Stoke Court, Stoke Poges, Slough SL2 4LY.

3.6.9 Self-monitoring – (ii) Home blood glucose monitoring

Various firms produce literature, audio-visual aids, and demonstrations to illustrate the use of their own meters and the glucose measuring strips. These may be obtained from the firms in question, e.g. Glucometer – Ames Corporation, Miles Laboratories Ltd. Ames Division, PO Box 37, Stoke Court, Stoke Poges, Slough SL2 4LY, UK.
Hypoguard Ltd., Dock Lane, Melton, Woodbridge, Suffolk IP12

IPE, UK.
Medistron Ltd., 6 Lawson-Hunt Industrial Park, Broadridge Heath, Horsham, West Sussex RH12 3JR, UK.
Reflolux – BCL, Bell Lane, Lewes, E. Sussex BN7 1LG, UK.

3.6.10 Computer based teaching/assessment programmes

1. *Diabetes* (cassette) Martin Dunitz Ltd., suitable for use with a simple computer (e.g. Sinclair Spectrum).
2. Ames Diabetes Management System (discs):
   Diabetes Education : ten interactive computer lessons for both IDDM and NIDDM at all levels with colour graphics and assessment facility. This program uses an IBM PC or IBM look-alike microcomputer which may also be used for *Clinic Management* (a patient record system) and *Patient Management* (the Ames Glucofacts Programme for use with the Ames Glucometer-M – a memory Glucometer).

3.6.11 Diabetes mini clinic

Produced by: Servier Laboratories Ltd., Windmill Road, Fulmer, Slough, SL3 6HH.
Package contains:

- Recall and follow-up sheet.
- Eye examination follow-up notes.
- Care of the feet guide.
- Transfer to GP care booklet.
- Diabetic identification cards.
- Ideal weight guide.
- Home testing diary.
- Dietary advice guide.
- Diabetes record card (patient).
- What is diabetes?
- Query card.
- Objective card.
- Insulin dose card.
- Test strip folder.
- Prescription request card.

REFERENCES AND FURTHER READING

Beaser, S.B. (1956) Teaching the diabetic patient. *Diabetes*, **5**, 146–9.

Brewin, T.B. (1985) Trust, truth and paternalism. *Lancet*, **ii**, 490.

Day, J. *Minimal Educational Facilities Report*. British Diabetic Association, London (10 Queen Anne Street, London W1M 0BD).

Etzwiler, D.D. and Sines, L.K. (1962) Juvenile diabetes and its management: family, social and academic implications, *J. Am. Med. Assoc.*, **181**, 304–8.

McCulloch, D.K., Mitchell, R.D., Ambler, J. and Tattersall, R.B. (1983) Influence of imaginative teaching of diet on compliance and metabolic control in insulin dependent diabetes, *Br. Med. J.*, **287**. 1858–61.

Mann, N.P. and Johnston, D.I. (1982) Total glycosylated haemoglobin levels in diabetic children. *Arch. Dis. Child.*, **57**, 434.

Miller, L.V. and Goldstein, J. (1972) More efficient care of diabetic patients in a county-hospital setting. *N. Engl. J. Med.*, **286**, 1388–91.

Miller, L.V., Goldstein, J. and Nicolaisen, G. (1978) Evaluation of patient's knowledge of diabetes self care. *Diabetes Care*, **1**, 275–80.

Tattersall, R.B. and McCulloch, D.K. (1984) Modern aspects of conventional insulin therapy. *Ann. Clin. Res.*, **16**, 107–17.

· Four ·

The control of blood glucose concentration

4.1 INTRODUCTION

The attempt to maintain blood glucose levels within the limits of normality (i.e. normoglycaemia) is an important part of the total management of the diabetic. However, the patient must be treated as a whole person and not as a 'blood glucose concentration' or 'a disease'. There is now good evidence to suggest that the maintenance of normal or near-normal glycaemia will delay the development of long-term complications and may even prevent them. Microvascular disease is rarely if ever seen in carbohydrate intolerance (i.e. blood glucose concentrations of greater than 6.7 mmol/1 but less than 10 mmol/1 (120–200 mg%) 2 hours after a 75 g glucose load). However, there is an increased incidence of macrovascular disease with this degree of carbohydrate intolerance.

The problems of persuading human beings to take action today because of what might happen in the future is a difficult one. The younger the patient the further off the future seems. Tomorrow never comes. From the outset, therefore, education and motivation is vital. A pattern of behaviour set in the earlier stages of the disease may be difficult to change later on. It is important to stress the positive aspects of good blood glucose control with good health today and the happy spin-off of good health tomorrow. If we are to convince the patient, it is important to set out the aims of treatment precisely.

4.2 THE AIMS OF TREATMENT

The aims of treatment are as follows:

1. A fit and happy patient.
2. A normal or near normal life style.

3. Normal or near normal blood glucose concentration.
4. No significant hypoglycaemia.

The aim is to produce a fit and happy patient leading a full and near normal life. The patient should have a normal or near-normal blood glucose concentration for most of the day and be free of significant hypoglycaemia. By achieving this degree of long-term glycaemic control, particularly when coupled with other measures such as 'taking a healthy diet', taking plenty of exercise, and not smoking, it is hoped to delay or even prevent the long-term complications of diabetes.

It is, however, worth considering the order in which these aims are set out. There is little point in striving for rigid normoglycaemia if it produces years of obsessional misery.

4.3 DESIRABLE STANDARDS OF CONTROL

Realistic goals for glycaemic control should be set. Both doctor and patient then know what they are hoping to achieve. Success will depend on many factors. Some of these are:

1. Patient's intelligence, social background, educational background, parental and family attitudes.
2. The stability of the family life. Marriage.
3. Initial diabetic education and instilled attitudes and motivation.
4. Type of work, its regularity, shift work.
5. Residual islet cell function.

The most important of these must be patient motivation and determination to achieve good glycaemic control. Many factors such as the patient's intelligence, educational background, social and family background, the environmental and personality are uninfluenced by the efforts of the health care team. High intelligence does not necessarily guarantee good control. Some of the worst patients to manage in this respect are doctors, nurses and solicitors! However, good diabetic education giving the correct start to the diabetic life and fostering the correct attitude is all important. It is for this reason that a whole chapter of this book is devoted to diabetic education.

Table 4.1 sets out the desirable standards of control. If it appears that the standards are set too high this is because in the past rather low standards have been set particularly for those patients treated with diet or diet with an oral hypoglycaemic agent. If the goals set out above are not obtainable with dietary treatment alone then the patient should be given an oral hypoglycaemic agent. If this fails to control glycaemia then the patient should be treated with insulin. Failure to comply with dietary advice should prompt caution particularly when adding to oral hypoglycaemic therapy and even more so when converting to insulin therapy. The dietary non-compliant patient will simply become increasingly obese when treated with oral hypoglycaemic agents or insulin.

Immediately following the diagnosis of insulin dependent diabetes there is often an initial period of good diabetic control. This is called 'the honeymoon period'. The standard of glycaemic control then gradually deteriorates particularly during adolescence. It may then be necessary to use multiple injection techniques or even

Table 4.1 Desirable standards of control.
'Good control' is all that we can hope for and suggested standards for this are indicated below. Ideal control is of course normoglycaemia 24 hours of a day. At present this is impossible to maintain in most cases.

		Blood test (mmol/, mg%)			
Type of diabetes	*Treatment*	*FBG*	*2 hr IBG*	*PP. BG*	*Urine glucose*
NIDD	Diet	3–5 (54–90)	3–7 (54–126)	3–7 (54–126)	0%
NIDD	Diet OHA	3–5 (54–90)	3–10 (54–180)	3–7 (54–126)	0%
IDD/ NIDD	Insulin	3–7 (54–126)	3–11 (54–198)	3–7 (54–126)	0–½%

NIDD = Non insulin dependent diabetes.
IDD = Insulin dependent diabetes.
FBG = Fasting blood glucose.
2 hr IBG = Blood glucose 2 hrs after the start of a meal.
PPBG = Preprandial blood glucose.
OHA = Oral hypoglycaemic agents – sulphonylurea or metformin.
With increasing age standards of control may be relaxed.
During adolescence, instability is often the rule.
The ideal is rarely achieved.
Weight should be steady in the adult and near to that which is ideal for patient's age, height and sex.
HbAl should be within the normal range.

continuous subcutaneous insulin infusion. However, poor control is often due to the problems of growing up and manipulation by the young person. This must be accepted as part of growing up. The aim should be not to alienate the patient in the hope that with maturity attitudes and control will improve.

With increasing age standards of glycaemic control may be relaxed. This should not be used as an excuse for sloppy management by the health care team. It is only too easy to regard the lack of positive health in an elderly person as being due to 'your age'. However, it must be remembered that the danger of hypoglycaemia outweighs the danger of long-term effects of modest hyperglycaemia (10–12 mmol/1, 180–216 mg%).

No matter whether the patient is insulin dependent or non insulin dependent the whole edifice of good glycaemic control is built on a sound foundation of dietary advice.

4.4 DIETARY ADVICE FOR THE DIABETIC

R.D. Hill and E. Robinson (Chief Dietitian, Poole General Hospital)

In the days before the discovery of insulin, diabetes was treated by severe dietary restriction. Patients literally starved to death. This restrictive practice continued even after the discovery of insulin and later of oral hypoglycaemic agents. Carbohydrates, when digested, produce glucose which when absorbed causes a rise in blood glucose concentration – ergo restrict carbohydrates and the problem is reduced. Life is never as simple as this. It was later discovered that severe restriction of carbohydrate intake actually made carbohydrate intolerance worse!

A restricted carbohydrate intake also brings problems. If carbohydrate is restricted, calorie intake must be made up by an intake of either fat or protein, or both. Foods containing mostly fat and protein tend to be low in bulk and may be consumed in excessive quantities to satisfy the appetite. Two serious consequences may stem from this. The excessive calorie intake produces weight gain and even obesity. The excessive fat intake produces hyperlipidaemia. In addition to this the patient may smoke in order to curb the appetite and prevent further weight gain. Obesity, hyperlipidaemia and smoking are important risk factors for macrovascular disease, particularly when coupled with hypertension and diabetes. The

Table 4.2 How diet has changed. Results are given as percentages of energy intake

	Carbohydrate	*Fat*	*Protein*
1920	10–20	60–80	10–20
1940	40	40–45	15–20
1980	50–55	30–35	15–20

consideration of these factors has led to a major revision of dietary ideas in the last decade.

Table 4.2 demonstrates the changing pattern of dietary advice during the last 60–70 years. From severe carbohydrate restriction we have moved to a diet rich in carbohydrate but reduced in fat.

What *Table 4.2* does not demonstrate is the major change in advice given with respect to the type of carbohydrate in the diet and its fibre content.

Monosaccharides (e.g. glucose and fructose in fruit juice) and disaccharides (e.g. lactose in milk) are rapidly digested, absorbed, and tend to cause a rapid but short-lived rise in blood glucose. Complex polysaccharides that are rich in fibre, are slowly digested, slowly absorbed, and cause a moderate rise in blood glucose concentration over a more prolonged period of time. This helps to prevent rapid swings in blood glucose concentration. Diets rich in fibre also reduce the cholesterol concentration in the blood and bring other benefits common to all whether diabetic or not. Thus the bowel function is improved and there is a possible reduction in the incidence of colonic neoplasms, gall stones and even varicose veins!

Having reviewed a few of the theoretical considerations behind modern dietary advice for the diabetic, the following general principles are suggested:

1. Take a limited dietary history and try to modify existing diets rather than attempt a total change in the patient's pattern of eating.
2. Aim for a total energy intake (calories) to maintain the patient's body weight within the norms set for the patient's age, sex and height. With respect to energy intake it is worth remembering (and reminding the patient) that to lose a mere one pound (0.5 kg)

of weight per week it is necessary to eat 500 calories per day less than that necessary to maintain a steady body weight. This is a sobering thought.
3. Do not restrict unrefined carbohydrate intake. The patient should ingest 50–55% of the calorie intake as carbohydrate.
4. Remove all monosaccharides and as many disaccharides from the diet as is possible and replace them with complex polysaccharides with a high fibre content.
5. Advise a diet low in total fat with polyunsaturated fats in preference to saturated fats.
6. Remember that our ability to change a patient's life-long eating habits is limited. Studies have shown that compliance with dietary advice is poor. The advice should be simple with attainable objectives.
7. The dietary advice given is not 'a diabetic diet' but sound advice for everyone – a diet for healthy living whether diabetic or not.

To help the health care team give necessary advice the section that follows attempts to relate the theoretical considerations given above to real foods.

For first-aid advice see section 2.3. A simplified large type version of dietary advice should be available for the elderly.

4.4.1 Dietary advice for patients with diabetes

(This advice is provided by the East Dorset Health Care District in the form of a small red booklet given to all patients with diabetes and complements the diabetic education sessions.)

(a) Introduction

The aim of your diet is to achieve good diabetic control, maintain an ideal weight and keep you fit and well.

The diabetic diet is a healthy way of eating for all the family and not just for the diabetic.

In the diet, a balance has to be achieved between the carbohydrate, fat and protein containing foods. The carbohydrate foods are especially important as they directly affect the blood sugar and so must be taken in controlled amounts (exchanges) to balance the blood sugar. At the same time, protein and fat intake must be considered as these foods provide calories and the total calorie intake affects diabetic control.

(b) Food to avoid

These foods should not be eaten as they contain too much sugar and would cause your blood sugar to rise above normal limits:

- Sugar, glucose, jam, marmalade, honey, syrup, treacle.
- Cakes, buns, sweet biscuits, and pastries containing sugar.
- Sweets and chocolates.
- Fruit tinned in syrup, jellies, tinned and instant puddings containing sugar.
- Drinks sweetened with sugar or glucose: squashes, Lucozade, lemonade, etc
- Sweet pickles and chutneys.
- Sweeteners containing sugar, e.g. Sucron, Twin Sugar.

(c) Foods containing little or no carbohydrate

These foods when eaten in normal amounts do not directly affect the blood sugar, but foods that contain protein and fat have an indirect effect on diabetic control. These foods, because of their calorie content must be taken in controlled amounts if you are overweight (see later).

(d) Food containing mostly protein

The following should be taken in moderation only, as they contain visible and invisible fat:

- Meat: Beef, lamb, mutton, veal, pork, ham, liver, kidney, heart, bacon, game. Chicken, turkey and rabbit have a low fat content and can be eaten in larger amounts.
- Fish: Herrings, kippers, mackerel, sardines, tuna, salmon, shellfish. All white fish (including smoked varieties) have a low fat content and can be eaten in larger amounts.
- Eggs.
- Cheese: All types. Edam, Camembert and Brie contain less fat, as do *Shape* and *Tendale*. Cottage cheese is very low in fat and can be eaten in large amounts.

In moderation means two or three helpings of the following each day.

Portion sizes:

- Meat 2–3 oz (50–75 g)
- Fish 3–4 oz (75–100 g)

- Cheese 2 oz (50 g) – once a day only
- Eggs 1 – once a day only

(e) Fatty foods

The following should be kept to an *absolute minimum*:

- Lard, dripping, suet, oils, cream.
- Butter/margarine 4–6 oz (100–150 g) per week, or
- Low fat spread – e.g. *Gold, Outline* – 8–12 oz (200–300 g) per week.

You should also:

1. Grill rather than fry your food.
2. Trim off any visible fat from meat.
3. Skim of any fat during cooking.
4. Pour off cream from milk before use or use skimmed milk.
5. Foods high in fat – e.g. pies, sausages, paté, diabetic chocolate, avocado pears, nuts – should be kept to a minimum.

(f) Freely allowed foods

N.B. The foods in italics contain some carbohydrate. These foods if eaten in large amounts must be counted in your carbohydrate allowance. See exchange list.

VEGETABLES. Artichokes, asparagus, aubergines, bean sprouts, *broad beans*, broccoli, brussels sprouts, cabbage, carrots, cauliflower, celery, courgettes, french beans, leeks, marrow, mushrooms, olives, onions, peppers, pumpkin, runner beans, spinach, swede, turnip, peas (fresh and frozen).

SALAD VEGETABLES. Vegetables, salad vegetables and fruits are sources of fibre especially when skins and pips are eaten.

Beetroot, cress, cucumber, lettuce, mustard, parsley, radishes, spring onions, tomatoes, watercress.

FRUITS. Blackberries, blackcurrants, gooseberries, *half grapefruit*, lemons, loganberries, olives, redcurrants, rhubarb.

SUNDRIES. Tea, coffee, water, clear soup, Oxo, Bovril, Marmite, soda water, diabetic and sugar free drinks and minerals, *tomato juice*.

Non-sugar sweeteners: saccharine, e.g. Sweetex, Hermesetas, Natrena, aspartame, e.g. Canderel.

Pepper, mustard, herbs, spices, vinegar, may be taken as required. Salt should be used in small amounts only.

If you need to lose weight, do not take fried and fatty foods, sorbitol, diabetic products (except diabetic squash), alcohol, especially diabetic beers and lagers. These all contain a large number of calories.

(g) Carbohydrate exchanges

All foods listed contain 10 g carbohydrate in the quantities indicated.

10 g carbohydrate = 1 exchange = 1 line = 1 standard portion

Use this list to vary the foods you eat while keeping to your prescribed amount of carbohydrate.

NOTES

1. All spoonfuls are level unless otherwise indicated.
2. The foods printed in **bold type** indicate foods that contain fibre.

Why is fibre important? Your diet should be high in fibre as this helps diabetic control. This works because fibre rich carbohydrate foods are digested and absorbed in a much smoother and slower way.

Take plenty of the fibre rich foods (shown in bold type) — ensure that you have at least one of these foods at each meal and snack.

Food	*Handy measure = 10 g carbohydrate*
BREAD AND BISCUITS	
Bread	
white	½ large slice – medium cut loaf
brown	⅔ large slice – thin cut loaf
wholemeal	1 small slice – thin cut loaf
Bread rolls	1 small bridge roll
	½ morning roll
Crispbreads	**2 Ryvita**
	2 Cracottes
	2 Krackerbread
Biscuits	**1 large digestive**
	1½ oatcakes
	1 bran biscuit
	2 cream crackers

Food	*Handy measure = 10 g carbohydrate*
2 water biscuits	
	2 plain, e.g. Rich Tea, Marie 5 Cheddars
BREAKFAST CEREALS	
All Bran	5 tablespoons
Bran Buds	4 tablespoons
Bran Flakes	4 tablespoons
Weetabix or similar cereal	1 biscuit
Weetaflakes	4 tablespoons
Puffed Wheat	15 tablespoons
Shredded Wheat	$\frac{2}{3}$ biscuit
Cornflakes	5 tablespoons
Muesli (unsweetened)	2 tablespoons
Spoonsize Shreddies	12
Special K	8 tablespoons
Rice Krispies	6 tablespoons
Raw oats or oatmeal	3 tablespoons
Porridge made with water	4 tablespoons
DRY CEREALS	
Custard powder, cornflour	1 tablespoon
Barley	1 tablespoon
Sago, tapioca, semolina	2 teaspoons
Flour	
white	$1\frac{1}{2}$ tablespoons
wholemeal	2 tablespoons
Soya flour	
low fat	9 tablespoons
full fat	14 tablespoons
Soya granules	13 tablespoons
Rice, **brown,** white	1 tablespoon
Spaghetti	
wholemeal	20 short (10″) strands
white	6 long (19″) strands
Lentils	2 tablespoons
COOKED CEREALS	
Rice, boiled – **brown,** white	2 tablespoons
Lentils, boiled	4 tablespoons
Chapatis – **wholemeal,** white	1 small teaplate size

Food	*Handy measure = 10 g carbohydrate*
VEGETABLES	
Potatoes	
boiled	1 egg sized
jacket	1 egg sized
roast*	1 egg sized
mashed	1 scoop
chips*	4–5 average
Beans – broad, boiled	10 tablespoons
dried, raw, all types	2 tablespoons
baked, in tomato sauce	4 tablespoons
Peas – tinned, marrowfat processed	7 tablespoons
dried, all types, raw	2 tablespoons
Parsnips	1 small
Sweetcorn, tinned, frozen	5 tablespoons
on the cob	½ medium cob
Beetroot (whole)	2 small
FRUITS	
Fresh	
Apple, peach, pear	1 medium sized
Apricots	3 medium
Banana	1 small
Cherries	12
Figs	1
Grapefruit	1 very large
Grapes	10
Mango	⅓ large one
Melon – all types	1 very large slice
Nectarines	1
Oranges	1 large
Pineapple	1 thick slice
Plums, dessert	2 large
Pomegranate	1 small
Raspberries	12 tablespoons
Strawberries	15 medium
Tangerines	2 large
Stewed	
Apples without sugar	6 tablespoons
Plums without sugar	4 medium

Food	*Handy measure = 10 g carbohydrate*
Dried	
Apricots	4 small
Currants, raisins, sultanas	2 tablespoons
Dates	3 small
Figs	1
Prunes	2 large
NUTS	
Peanuts*	100 g packet
DAIRY PRODUCTS	
Milk, skimmed or fresh	1 glass or ⅓ pint
Evaporated, unsweetened	6 tablespoons
Yoghurt	
plain	1 small carton
ordinary fruit	½ small carton
sugar free fruit	1 small carton
Ice cream, plain	1 scoop or brickette
BEVERAGES	
Natural fruit juices, unsweetened	
Apple, pineapple	6 tablespoons (3 fl oz)
Orange	7 tablespoons (3½ fl oz)
Grapefruit	8 tablespoons (4 fl oz)
Tomato	1 large glass (9 fl oz)
Horlicks, Bournvita, Ovaltine	2 heaped teaspoons
MISCELLANEOUS	
Sausages*	2 large, 3 thin, 4 chipolatas*
Fish fingers	2
Soup, cream	1 cup
Scotch egg	1

* Indicates high fat foods.

(h) Sample diet

			Carbohydrate exchanges from list
Breakfast			
e.g. Half-grapefruit			
Egg or bacon			
Tomato, mushrooms etc.	and		.... Exchanges
Tea, coffee		e.g.	
Mid-morning			
e.g. Tea, coffee, Oxo, Bovril	and		.... Exchanges
		e.g.	
Midday meal			
e.g. Meat or fish or cheese or	and		.... Exchanges
egg, vegetables, salad		e.g.	
Mid-afternoon			
e.g. Tea, coffee	and		.... Exchanges
		e.g.	
Evening meal			
e.g. Meat or fish or cheese or	and		.... Exchanges
egg, vegetables, salad		e.g.	
Bed time			
e.g. Tea, coffee, Oxo, Bovril	and		.... Exchanges
		e.g.	
	Total exchanges		

Always take the stated number of exchanges at each meal and use the exchange list to vary your choice of carbohydrate foods.

NB. The person advising this patient completes the number of carbohydrate exchanges allowed for each meal and adds examples for each meal.

(i) Diet during illness

For diabetics taking insulin or tablets.

During illness you must continue taking your insulin or tablets. You must therefore take your usual amount of carbohydrate. At such times more concentrated forms of carbohydrate may be used if you are unable to manage solid food.

Examples of fluids to give:

ONE EXCHANGE

1. 7 fl oz milk ($\frac{1}{3}$ pint or a glassful).
2. 2 fl oz Lucozade.
3. 7 tablespoons unsweetened orange juice ($3\frac{1}{2}$ fl oz).
4. 8 tablespoons unsweetened grapefruit juice (4 fl oz).
5. 2 heaped teaspoons glucose in diabetic squash.
6. 2 level teaspoons sugar in diabetic squash.
7. 2 oz ice cream (1 brickette)
8. 1 carton natural yoghurt.
9. Egg custard using 7 fl oz milk.
10. 1 cup thickened soup.

TWO EXCHANGES

1. 7 fl oz milk and 2 heaped teaspoons of Ovaltine or Horlicks.
2. 7 fl oz milk and 2 heaped teaspoons of glucose.
3. 7 fl oz milk and 2 level teaspoons of sugar.
4. 7 fl oz milk and $\frac{2}{3}$ oz (3 level tablespoons) of Complan powder.
5. 4 fl oz Lucozade.
6. 7 tablespoons unsweetened orange juice ($3\frac{1}{2}$ fl oz) and 2 level teaspoons of sugar.
7. 7 fl oz milk and 2 oz ice cream whisked together as milk shake.
8. Milk pudding using $\frac{1}{2}$ oz cereal and 7 fl oz milk.
9. ½ packet Carnation Build Up and 7 fl oz milk.

THREE EXCHANGES

1. 1 oz ($4\frac{1}{2}$ level tablespoons) Complan and $\frac{1}{2}$ pint milk.
2. 2 heaped teaspoons Ovaltine or Horlicks and 7 fl oz milk and 2 level teaspoons of sugar.
3. 1 carton of ordinary fruit yoghurt and 2 level teaspoons sugar.
4. 15 mls (3 teaspoons) Ribena, 7 fl oz milk and 2 oz ice cream whisked together as a milk shake.

FOUR EXCHANGES

1. 1 packet of Carnation Build Up and ½ pint milk.
2. 1 oz ($4\frac{1}{2}$ level tablespoons) Complan and $\frac{1}{2}$ pint milk and 2 level teaspoons sugar.
3. 30 ml (6 teaspoons) Ribena, 7 fl oz milk and 2 oz ice cream.
4. 1 medium banana, $\frac{1}{2}$ pint milk, 2 oz ice cream whisked together as a milk shake.

(j) Alcohol

You should consult your doctor before including any alcohol in your diet if you are taking insulin or tablets, as alcohol directly affects your blood sugar level. Alcoholic drinks with a high sugar content should be avoided (e.g. sweet wines, sweet sherries, and liqueurs). Other alcohol drinks should be limited to a maximum of 2–3 units per day.

One unit is equal to:

Dry wine –	1 small glass
Dry sherry –	1 small glass
Dry Vermouth –	1 small glass
Spirits –	1 single measure
Beer/lager/cider –	$\frac{1}{2}$ pint

Add only water, soda water and sugar-free mixers.

Avoid ordinary tonic water, bitter lemon, ginger ale, and lemonade.

Remember:

1. The carbohydrate content of alcoholic drinks should not be counted in your daily carbohydrate allowance. You must not substitute alcohol for your normal carbohydrate intake.
2. Low carbohydrate beers, lagers and ciders should be avoided as they have a high alcohol and calorie content.
3. It is important to avoid food and drink with a high sugar content when drinking alcohol i.e. mixers must be sugar free. Food should accompany or follow the consumption of alcohol. This will minimise the risk of hypoglycaemia in those taking insulin or tablets. The possibility of hypoglycaemia persists at least 4 hours after alcohol has been taken.
4. Do not take any alcohol if you are overweight.

(k) Special diabetic products

These are expensive and not an essential part of your diet. Please ask the dietitian before taking them. Diabetic biscuits, cakes, and chocolates are not freely allowed as they contain carbohydrate and so must be counted as part of your carbohydrate allowance. See packet for details (10 g available carbohydrate = 1 exchange). Do not take these products if you are overweight.

4.5 Oral hypoglycaemic agents

Non insulin dependent diabetics who fail to achieve the desired standard of glycaemic control as indicated in *Table 4.1* on diet alone should be considered for treatment with an oral hypoglycaemic agent. In general oral hypoglycaemic agents should not be used until a period of dietary treatment has been tried for 2–3 months. Adherence to the diet may be assessed by measuring the patient's weight. In obesity, failure to lose weight may suggest either poor dietary compliance or that the patient has been given too many calories in the diet. On the other hand, the maintenance of normal weight with improved glycaemic control suggests good compliance with dietary advice.

Oral hypoglycaemic agents fall into two broad groups. These are the sulphonylureas and the biguanides:

1. Sulphonylureas and related drugs:

Acetohexamide	(Dimelor)
Chlorpropamide	(Diabenese, Melitase)
Glibenclamide	(Daonil, Euglucon, Diabeta)
Glibornuride	(Glutril)
Gliclazide	(Diamicron)
Glipizide	(Glibenese, Minodiab, Glucotrol)
Gliquidone	(Glurenorm)
Glymidine	(Gondafon)
Tolazamide	(Tolanase)
Tolbutamide	(Pramidex, Rastinon, Mellinese)

2. Biguanides:

Metformin	(Glucophage)

(a) Sulphonylureas

The precise mode of action of sulphonylureas is still not completely understood. However, there is some evidence that in the early stages at least sulphonylureas stimulate pancreatic production of insulin. In addition to this they also appear to increase the number of insulin receptors and to some extent affect platelet adherence. The relevance of platelet adherence to vascular disease is as yet unknown. When prescribing sulphonylureas the following points should be considered:

1. In obesity due to non-dietary compliance, sulphonylureas simply

reduce blood glucose levels, reduce glycosuria, and therefore retain calories. The net result is a steady increase in weight and further insulin resistance. (Precisely the same argument may be used against using insulin in obesity.)

2. Chlorpropamide is a long-acting drug. It may cause severe hypoglycaemia in the elderly. In addition to this chlorpropamide is known to cause fluid retention which may precipitate heart failure in the elderly. It is not advisable to give chlorpropamide to patients over the age of 60 years.
3. Tolbutamide is a short-acting drug which has the disadvantage of requiring twice or thrice daily dosage. Patients often forget to take the second or third dose. However, dangerous hypoglycaemia is unlikely and fluid retention is not a problem.
4. Gliquidone is a short-acting compound which has to be taken three times a day. This compound has the advantage that its action is not affected by renal failure and it may therefore be used with benefit in this situation.
5. It is sensible to get to know a given sulphonylurea and learn to use it safely and effectively. Glibenclamide and gliclazide are the drugs of choice. They have been found to be effective and safe. With glibenclamide the starting dose is 2.5 mg per day. It is a simple matter to ask a patient to increase the dose by an increment of 2.5 mg per day at four day intervals. The dose should be increased every four days until glycosuria disappears or until a maximum dose of 10 mg twice daily is reached. Gliclazide may be similarly used with a starting dose of 40 mg per day. Increments of 40 mg daily should be added at four day intervals until glycosuria disappears or a maximum dose of 320 mg per day is reached. The larger dose should be taken in divided doses. By using this simple regime for both glibenclamide and gliclazide hypoglycaemic reactions may be avoided. Gliclazide is said to cause less weight gain and less hypoglycaemia than glibenclamide. After 2 months freedom from glycosuria the blood sugar and HbA1 should be assessed. If the desired standard of control has not been reached then a further increase in dose should be given and a reassessment made 3 months later.

Side effects of treatment with sulphonylureas. The sulphonylurea group of drugs is now widely used. Experience has shown that side effects are infrequent and not severe. Facial flushing may be a problem after taking alcohol particularly with chlorpropamide. This may be distressing but the patient should be reassured for it is not dangerous.

Anorexia, nausea, vomiting, epigastric discomfort and occasional diarrhoea are also seen.

In the nervous system, weakness and paraesthesia have been described.

Rarely photosensitivity affects the skin but other allergic reactions are perhaps more common.

Jaundice, eosinophilia and fever have also been described.

It is important to realize that cross-reaction between one sulphonylurea and another is very common. The reaction shown to one compound will almost certainly be produced by another.

If the desirable standard of control is not achieved with good dietary compliance and the addition of sulphonylurea then the addition of a biguanide or conversion to insulin treatment must be considered.

(b) Biguanides

Biguanides reduce blood glucose by stimulating non insulin dependent peripheral glucose metabolism. Both insulin and sulphonylureas not only lower the blood glucose concentration but also reduce the concentration of other abnormal metabolites towards those concentrations found in the non-diabetic. However, the biguanides tend to increase the concentration of lactate and do not return other abnormal metabolites towards normal levels. In the presence of renal or hepatic dysfunction or in a situation of high lactate production (e.g. severe hypotension in myocardial infarction), lactate levels may rise sufficiently to produce marked lactic acidosis. Coma in lactic acidosis has a mortality of 50%. Before prescribing a biguanide these factors must be considered carefully. The first biguanide to be marketed was Phenformin. This has been withdrawn from the UK market because of the danger of lactic acidosis. Metformin does not appear to carry the same risk but should be used in selected patients only. These are usually obese subjects failing to reach the desirable standards of control on diet, or who gain weight on sulphonylureas. In this respect metformin has the advantage that it produces a degree of anorexia! It is important to ensure that the patient has normal hepatic and renal function before prescribing metformin. The dose of metformin hydrochloride is

500 mg every 8 hours or 850 mg every 12 hours.

The most significant side effects of biguanide therapy are those affecting the gastrointestinal tract. Anorexia, nausea, vomiting and diarrhoea are the most prominent.

Patients who fail to reach the desired standard of control on diet and oral hypoglycaemic agents should be treated with insulin.

4.6 TREATMENT WITH INSULIN

4.6.1 Introduction

In the non-diabetic state blood glucose concentrations are kept within a narrow band of normality. This glucose homeostasis is achieved by a complex interplay of several factors. Feeding, glucagon secretion and stress (catecholamine and cortisol secretion) all tend to increase blood glucose concentrations. Any tendency for the blood glucose to rise is immediately counteracted by an increase in insulin secretion. The increase in insulin concentration switches off hepatic glucose production (from gluconeogenesis and glycogenolysis). The increased insulin concentration also stimulates peripheral glucose uptake. The net result is a fall in blood glucose concentration.

With fasting and on exercise blood glucose concentrations tend to fall. This is immediately associated with a decrease in insulin secretion. The fall in insulin concentration switches on hepatic glucose production and peripheral blood glucose uptake is diminished. This results in a net increase in blood glucose concentration and glucose homeostatsis is maintained. In addition to these homeostatic mechanisms, a fall in blood glucose concentration is counteracted by glucagon secretion. This stimulates hepatic glucose production and tends to raise the blood glucose level. Similarly the secretion of catecholamines and cortisol tend to raise the blood glucose concentration

It will be seen that in the non-diabetic there is a complex closed loop feedback system which reacts promptly to any tendency for the blood glucose to rise and fall (*Figures 4.1* and *4.2*).

In the diabetic the situation is very different. Following total pancreatectomy the patient is not only denied the benefits of insulin secretion but also loses glucagon secretion. There is thus a tendency for the blood glucose level to rise and fall rapidly and uncontrollably,

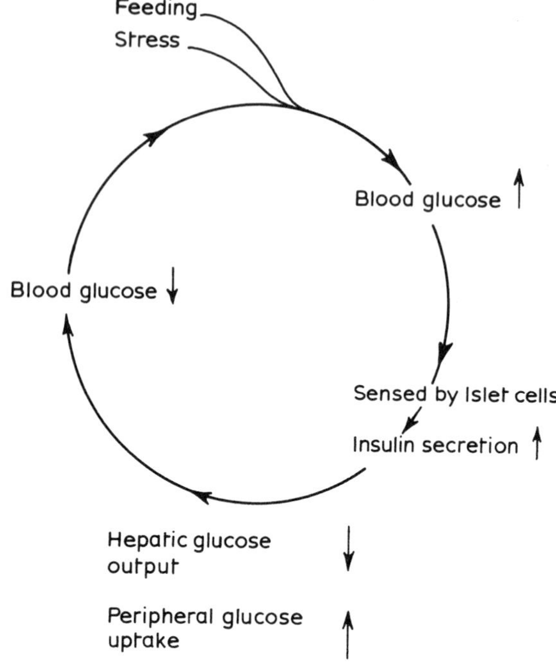

Figure 4.1 Glucose homeostasis feedback loop – response to a rise in blood glucose concentration.

and following this operation blood glucose is often very difficult to control.

As indicated in Chapter 1 the type of diabetes acquired by a patient will depend on residual islet cell function. Patients having near-normal islet cell function perhaps associated with obesity and insulin resistance will require only a diet to control blood glucose levels. Patients having diminished islet cell function but retaining enough insulin secretion to prevent ketoacidosis will manage on a diet with oral hypoglycaemic agents. However, when insulin secretion falls below a certain level then ketoacidosis develops and the patient becomes insulin dependent. Insulin-dependent diabetics may have some residual islet cell function or none at all. The ease with which blood glucose concentrations are controlled is to some extent dependent on how much insulin secretion the patient has.

In the non-diabetic the islet cells maintain a steady output of

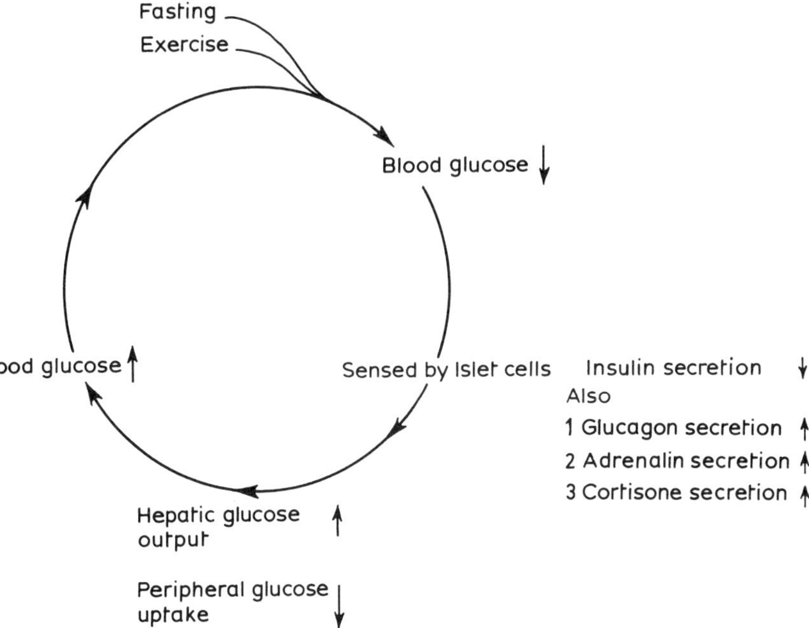

Figure 4.2 Glucose homeostasis feedback loop – response to a fall in blood glucose concentration.

insulin (background insulin secretion). In addition to this background secretion the islet insulin output is increased when blood glucose tends to rise (*Figure 4.1*). Thus after a meal there is a rapid rise in insulin secretion to counteract the effects of the meal. Ideally any therapeutic intervention in the insulin-deficient patient should attempt to mimic this situation. The main problem with giving insulin by injection is that once the injection is given there can be no switching on and off of insulin absorption. The ideal solution might appear to be pancreatic or islet cell transplantation. Unfortunately, the techniques have not yet reached a sufficient degree of reliability and safety to allow widespread application. Another possible solution is that of the implanted insulin infusion pump. Here a sensor detects blood glucose levels, supplies information to a miniature computer, which in turn supplies information to a pump. Insulin is pumped from a reservoir into a venous line preferably in the portal system. Again technology is not yet sufficiently advanced to make this a feasible technique for widespread use. However, consideration of this method of treatment does highlight one of the problems of insulin injected into the periphery. In order to obtain sufficient insulin concentrations in the portal system (to have the required effect on the liver) it is necessary to have very high peripheral insulin concentrations. There is some evidence that this is harmful and may be atherogenic.

The feed back loop shown in *Figures 4.1* and *4.2* demonstrates the complex nature of blood glucose control. Without effective insulin secretion the cycle of control is broken.

Having considered the various mechanisms of blood glucose homeostasis it is not surprising that some difficulty is often experienced with control of blood glucose levels by insulin injections. We have no closed loop feedback mechanism, and therefore once the injection is given we have no control over the absorption of the insulin and resultant insulin concentrations in the blood. It is perhaps more surprising that reasonable control can ever be achieved by this method.

Continuous subcutaneous insulin infusion of insulin (CSII) using a small portable insulin infusion pump attempts to mimic pancreatic secretion of insulin. A constant infusion of insulin (Neutral soluble or Human actrapid) is given at a rate of 12–24 units per 24 hours to maintain a background concentration of insulin. A bolus of 4–6 units is given three times each day with each main meal. The open loop mechanism without feedback is partially closed by home blood glucose monitoring. The patients adjust the background rate of insulin infusion by reference to the fasting blood glucose in the morning. Bolus injections are adjusted according to preprandial blood glucose concentrations.

Insulin pumps should be reserved for selected patients who are not controlled by other methods. These patients should be supervised by special centres experienced in the use of CS11. The technique is not without its dangers (hypoglycaemia, sudden onset ketoacidosis, see also Appendix 3).

A close second to CSII is the multiple injection technique (MIT) Here a long-acting insulin such as Human Ultratard is given in daily injections. Background insulin levels gradually rise and by the third day a steady state is reached. Bolus insulin is supplied by a short-acting insulin such as Human Actrapid or Neutral soluble given by an injection before each meal. This involves the patient giving three or four injections of insulin per day. The burden of frequent injections has been relieved to some extent by the development of simple instruments for injections such as the Novopen. (Plate 2). This instrument contains a cartridge of Actrapid insulin. The fountain-pen-like Novopen can be carried in the pocket and an injection given without any fuss at any time during the day. Adjustment of the insulin dose is made on the basis of the fasting and preprandial blood glucose concentrations as for CSII (see above).

Perhaps the most widely used and practical insulin regimen is the twice daily regimen using at each injection a mixture of a short-acting insulin and a longer acting insulin. This will be described in detail below.

The single daily injection of a long-acting insulin is the least successful method of insulin delivery. However, if the patient has a reasonable amount of residual islet cell function then this method can be quite successful in the control of blood glucose concentrations.

Whatever method is used for insulin delivery partial closure of the feedback loop may be obtained by careful home blood glucose monitoring.

When considering treatment with insulin the following questions need to be answered:

1. What are the indications for treatment with insulin?
2. How much insulin is required?
3. Which insulin regimen should be used?

4.6.2 Indications for insulin treatment

1. Hyperglycaemic precoma or coma with ketoacidosis.
2. Hyperglycaemic coma or precoma without ketoacidosis.
3. Insulin dependent diabetes.
4. Non insulin dependent diabetes not achieving an acceptable standard of control with diet and oral hypoglycaemic agents.

Indications 1 and 2 will be discussed in a later chapter (see Chaper 5).

4.6.3 How much insulin is required?

The total daily insulin requirement may be calculated (as a starting dose) by the simple formula 0.2–0.5 units per kilogram body weight per day.

If insulin is to be given as a twice daily regimen then two-thirds of the total daily dose should be given in the morning and one-third in the evening.

The ratio of the rapidly acting component (e.g. Human Actrapid or Neutral soluble) to the longer acting component (e.g. Human Monotard or Isophane) should be approximately one-third quick-acting insulin and two-thirds longer acting insulin.

The injection of insulin should be given approximately 10–20 minutes before a meal. Injections should be given subcutaneously.

4.6.4 Which insulin regimen?

The twice daily insulin regimen is probably the most satisfactory for the majority of patients. A few patients will manage on a single dose of insulin each day. It is likely that these are patients who have a considerable amount of residual islet cell function.

The choice of insulin regimen will determine the type of insulin(s) to be used. *Table 4.3* lists the bewildering number of insulins now available. They may be classified according to:

1. The species of origin (bovine/porcine/human).
2. Degree of purification and pH (purified /monocomponent/acid, neutral).
3. Duration of action.

The species of origin and purity of the insulin is important since repeated injections of foreign protein stimulate antibody production which binds the insulin. The advantages and disadvantages of having a circulating pool of bound insulin which is slowly released as free insulin concentration falls have been debated. Antibodies raised to impurities contained in insulin have, at least theoretically, possible dangers.

The older purified bovine and porcine insulins are being largely replaced by highly purified porcine insulins because of their decreased immunogenicity. However, even these insulins are now being replaced by biosynthetic insulin (produced by recombinant DNA technology, e.g. Lilly) or by enzymatically modified porcine insulins (e.g. Novo and Nordisk) having the structure of human insulin. It is important to reassure patients that these new insulins are not obtained from human material! The so called human insulins

Table 4.3 List of insulins. The strength of insulin to be dispensed must be stated in the prescription (i.e. U-20, U-40, U-80, or U-100, indicating the number of units per c.c.)

Purified (pH 3.2)	*Highly purified* (neutral)
(a) Short-acting insulin preparations	
Pork/bovine mixture:	Bovine origin:
Soluble insulin BP	Hypurin neutral (C.P.Pharm)
Regular insulin USP	Neusulin (Wellcome)
	Quicksol (Boots)
Regular Iletin I (Lilly)	Regular Iletin II (Lilly)
	Porcine origin:
	Velosulin (Nordisk)
	Human insulins:
	Human Actrapid (Novo)
	Novolin Toronto (Connaught-Novo)
	Novolin R (Squibb-Novo)
	Humulin S (Lilly), Humulin R (Lilly)
	Human Velosulin (Nordisk)
(b) Insulins of longer duration of action suitable for use with twice daily regimen when mixed with a short acting insulin	
Bovine origin:	Bovine origin (N.P.H. Type):
Isophane insulin injection (NPH)	Hypurin Isophane (C.P. Pharm)
	Neuphane (Wellcome)
	Monophane (Boots)
	NPH Iletin II (Bovine) (Lilly)
Bovine–porcine:	Porcine origin (N.P.H. Type):
Semilente Iletin I (Lilly)	Insulatard (Nordisk)
NPH Iletin I (Lilly)	NPH Iletin II (Porcine) (Lilly)
	Monocomponent insulins porcine origin:
	Semitard MC (Novo)
	Human insulins:
	Human Monotard (Novo)
	Novolin L (Squibb-Novo)
	NPH Type
	Human Protophane (Novo)
	Novolin N (Squibb-Novo)
	Novolin NPH (Connaught-Novo)
	Human Insulatard (Nordisk)
	Humulin I (Lilly), Humulin N (Lilly)

(c) Ready mixed insulins suitable for twice daily regimens when patients cannot or find difficulty in mixing their own insulins ('biphasic insulin')

Porcine/bovine mixture:

Rapitard MC (Novo). A mixure of crystalline bovine insulin and neutral porcine insulin. The mixture contains 25% of a short-acting component and 75% of the longer acting component.

Porcine mixtures:

Mixtard (Nordisk). Contains crystalline neutral highly purified insulins in a mixture having 30% of the insulin as a short-acting component and 70% as a long-acting component.

Initard (Nordisk). Also a mixture of highly purified isophane and neutral insulin but having 50% as the short-acting component and 50% as the long-acting component.

Human mixtures:

Human Mixtard 30/70 (Nordisk). Composition as for Mixtard but using human insulins.

Human Actraphane 30/70 (Novo) (30% H. Actrapid, 70% H. Isophane)

Human Initard 50/50 (Nordisk). Composition as for Initard but using human insulins.

Humulin M1 (Lilly). A mixture of 10% human soluble and 90% human isophane.

Humulin M2 (Lilly). A mixture of 20% human soluble and 80% human isophane.

(d) Insulin mixtures suitable for the once daily regimen

Containing a short-acting component (30%) and a long-acting component (70%). They all contain bovine insulin or a bovine/porcine insulin mixture:

Insulin Zinc suspension Lente (bovine)
Hypurin Lente (Weddel) (bovine)
Lentard MC (Novo) (bovine and porcine)
Neulente (Wellcome) (bovine)
Lente Iletin I (Lilly) (bovine and porcine)
Lente Iletin II (Lilly) (bovine and porcine)

Human insulin:

Humulin L (Lilly)

Neutral soluble insulin can be mixed with the above mixtures to increase the short-acting component. However, they must not be mixed with insulins having a pH of 3.

(e) Other insulins having long duration suitable for background insulin therapy in combination with short-acting insulins

Bovine origin:
Insulin zinc suspension (crystalline) Ultra Lente BP.
Tempulin (Boots).

Bovine–porcine origin:
Ultralente Iletin I (Lilly)

Human insulin:
Human Ultratard (Novo)

Note:
1. The varying composition of mixtures in respect of the proportion of short-acting and long-acting components.
2. Rapitard contains insulin of bovine origin and is not suitable if allergy to bovine insulin exists.

have little or no immunogenicity. If anything, the human insulins appear to act slightly more quickly and have a slightly shorter duration. With biosynthetic production, costs are likely to fall and this will almost certainly be the main reason for the change to the human type of insulins.

Many insulins are now available in strengths of 20, 40, 80 and 100 units per cc. In the United States, Canada, Australia, New Zealand and the United Kingdom, 100 unit strength (U-100) has been almost universally adopted. U-20, U-40, and U-80 insulins are still used in Europe. It is important to state the strength of insulin to be dispensed when prescribing insulin. It is also important to use the correct syringe calibrated to the insulin used.

Manufacturers of insulin produce charts showing the duration of insulin action. However, how long an insulin acts depends on many factors in addition to the type of insulin used. These factors include:

1. The size of the dose (volume injected).
2. The site of injection (rate of absorption).
3. Rate of destruction (slow in renal failure).
4. The presence of insulin binding proteins.

As with most forms of therapy it is better to become familiar with a few regimens and learn to use them safely and effectively. For this reason only three regimens will be described in detail.

4.6.5 The twice daily insulin regimen

1. Total units per day = 0.2–0.5 units per kilogram body weight.

2. Morning dose = ⅔rd of total daily dose.
3. Evening dose = ⅓rd of total daily dose.
4. Ratio of short-acting insulin to longer acting insulin, 1 : 2.
5. Time of injection = 10–20 minutes before a meal, given subcutaneously.
6. Suitable insulins. Short-acting insulins (see *Table 4.3 (a)*). Longer acting insulins (see *Table 4.3 (b)*).

Figure 4.3 is used as a teaching aid. It shows the patient how the twice daily regimen works and how the insulin components of the regimen may be altered in order to obtain blood glucose control without hypoglycaemia. A step-by-step explanation must be given to give the patient full understanding.

To monitor the effect of insulin therapy, blood glucose (home monitoring or laboratory) or post voided urine specimens must be

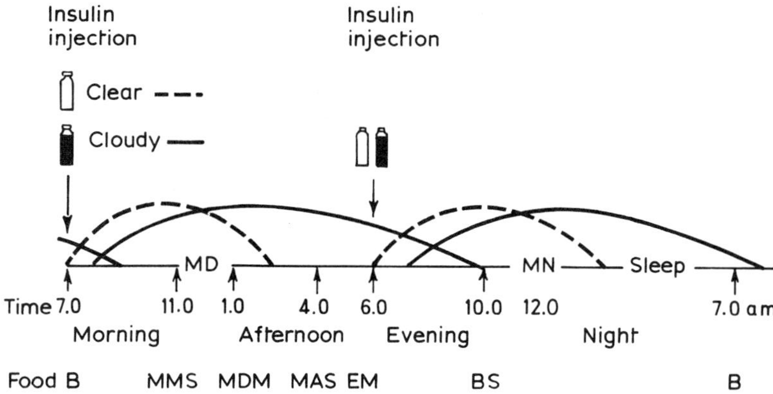

Figure 4.3 The twice daily insulin regimen. The horizontal line represents the time course throughout the day divided into periods as indicated, i.e. morning, afternoon, evening and night. MD = Midday; MN = Midnight. Below the horizontal line is indicated approximate meal times. B = Breakfast; MMS = Midmorning snack; MDM = Midday meal; MAS = Midafternoon snack; EM = Evening meal; BS = Bedtime snack. Below each mealtime the appropriate number of grams of carbohydrate taken may be written. Above the line is shown the time course and action of insulin injected. Injections of two insulins are given as a mixed dose before breakfast and before the evening meal. The more rapidly acting insulin (clear, i.e. Actrapid or Soluble) is shown by the dotted line and the more prolonged acting insulin (cloudy, i.e. Monotard or Isophane) is shown by the solid line.

taken before breakfast, before midday meal, before evening meal, and before retiring to bed.

The following advice should be given to patients to allow them to adjust their insulin dose:

1. Not more than 2–4 units should be added or subtracted in any one day at any one time.
2. Only one insulin should be adjusted at any one time.
3. Changes should be made gradually to allow adjustment throughout the day.
4. If a high blood glucose value or glycosuria is found in the fasting state then the evening 'cloudy' insulin (e.g. Monotard or Isophane insulins) should be increased. If a high blood glucose value or glycosuria is found before the evening meal then the morning 'cloudy' insulin should be increased. Similarly, if glycosuria or high blood glucose value is found before retiring to bed, then the evening 'clear' insulin (e.g. Actrapid or Soluble insulin) should be increased. A high blood glucose value or glycosuria occuring before midday would be an indication for an increase in the morning 'clear' insulin.
5. If hypoglycaemia is experienced during the morning then it is the morning 'clear' insulin which should be decreased. If hypoglycaemia occurs in the afternoon then it is the morning 'cloudy' insulin which should be decreased. Hypoglycaemia occurring in the evening or early night is an indication to reduce the evening 'clear' insulin and hypoglycaemia occurring during the night is an indication to reduce the evening 'cloudy' insulin.

By gradually adjusting the dose of insulin good control of the diabetes is usually possible. Fine tuning of the control and adjustment for exercise can be achieved by increasing or decreasing the carbohydrate intake at various times of the day.

A simple 'slide rule' (see inside back cover) based on the above has been developed by Sister P. Hindley (Poole Diabetic Liaison Sister) and marketed by Ames Division, Miles Laboratories Ltd., Stoke Poges, Slough SL2 4LY, England.

4.6.6 Single dose regimen

This regimen should not be used unless good control is achieved without hypoglycaemia and with a dose of less than 50 units per day.

It is most useful in patients who are fortunate enough to have significant residual islet cell function and who lead lives that do not require the flexibility of other regimens.

Insulin Zinc Suspension Lente or Lentard MC is the insulin of choice. It is given at a starting dose of 0.2–0.5 units per kilogram body weight per day.

The insulin is given subcutaneously 30 minutes before breakfast. The dose is increased by increments of 2–4 units per day until the urine tests show no glycosuria at some time during the day. The dose is then increased with the object of making the patient free of glycosuria at all times through the day without precipitating hypoglycaemia. This may be difficult on a single dose of insulin and it is usually necessary to adjust the quantity and timing of carbohydrate to avoid hypoglycaemia.

This regimen must be regarded as a second best and is not recommended except for patients with considerable residual islet cell function and in whom good control is achieved without difficulty.

4.6.7 Multiple injection technique

If the patient fails to attain adequate control with a twice daily regimen then the multiple injection technique may be applicable provided that it is acceptable from the patient's point of view. Here a steady state background insulin concentration is achieved by giving Human Ultratard daily. It takes 3 days to achieve a steady state and from then on the injection of Human Ultratard maintains a steady state or near steady state insulin concentration. On this background, boluses of a short acting insulin such as Human Actrapid or Neutral Soluble are given with each main meal (see *Figure 4.4*). Human Ultratard is given in a daily dose of 5–12 units either as a separate injection before going to bed or in combination with the third bolus with the evening meal. A quick acting insulin such as Human Actrapid or Neutral Soluble insulin is given in a bolus of 6–8 units on three occasions during the day before each main meal. The fasting blood glucose level is adjusted by adjusting the dose of Human Ultratard at 4 day intervals. The preprandial blood glucose level before the midday meal, before the evening meal, and the blood glucose before going to bed are adjusted by varying the relevant bolus of insulin as shown in *Figure 4.4*.

The multiple injection technique is made more bearable by using a

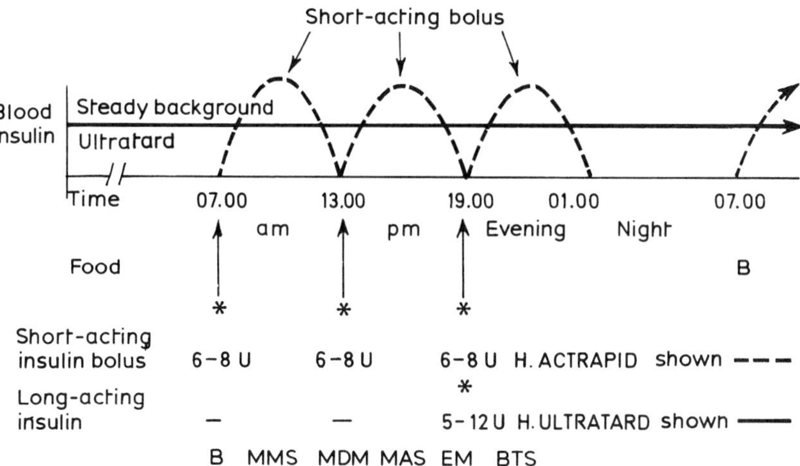

Figure 4.4 Multiple insulin injection regimen.

Novopen or similar instrument. This syringe delivers 2 units of Human Actrapid for each press of the plunger. The pen is loaded with an insulin cartridge (Human Actrapid – Novo) and this obviates the necessity for drawing up insulin and the routine involved.

If good control is not achieved with the multiple injection technique then continuous subcutaneous infusion of insulin (CSII) should be considered (see Appendix 3). This technique is not without its dangers. In the United States fatalities from hypoglycaemia have occurred. The technique should be used with selected cases only and should be used in centres experienced in the technique. Patients requiring this type of therapy should be referred to a special centre.

4.6.8 Special situations

(a) Patients with problems mixing insulins

Patients who are not able to mix their own insulins may be managed using biphasic insulins which consist of a fixed ratio mixture of a rapidly acting insulin and an intermediate acting insulin. Mixtard (Nordisk) contains crystalline neutral highly purified insulins in a mixture having 30% of insulin as a short-acting component and 70% as a long-acting component. Human insulin of this type is now available. Initard (Nordisk) is also a mixture of highly purified

Isophane and Neutral insulins having 50% as a short-acting component and 50% as a long-acting component. Using these mixed insulins in a twice daily regimen it is usually possible to get quite good control. Initard is particularly useful for those patients requiring a boost of short acting insulin in the 6 hours following the injection.

Fixed ratio insulin mixtures and the twice daily regimen is particularly useful in the elderly. A district nurse may draw up both the morning and evening dose of insulin into a syringe, give the morning dose, and leave the evening dose for the patient or a relative to give. It is possible to do this even with partially sighted people who are not able to draw up their own insulins.

(b) Blind or partially sighted diabetics

For blind or partially sighted diabetics the problems of insulin dose measurement is paramount. The 'click count' syringe (which has a ratchet mechanism making a click every time 2 units of insulin are drawn into the syringe) and the fixed dose syringes are useful. However, the adjustment of these syringes must be constantly checked as they tend to work loose and a variable dose may then be given by the patient.

4.6.9 Insulin syringes

It is essential to use the syringe which is appropriate to the strength of insulin used. They may be glass or disposable:

1. Glass syringes. BS1619/2, 0.5 ml (50 units) and 1.0 ml (100 units).
2. U-100 Disposable syringes. Several disposable syringes are now available in 0.5 ml (50 units) and 1.0 ml (100 units) sizes. The best of these syringes incorporate a very fine, sharp, short needle with a very low dead space. This is a distinct advantage when using insulin of high concentration (U-100) and mixing two different insulins together.

(a) Care of the syringe

Glass syringes need to be sterilized and stored in industrial spirit between injections. Suitable plastic spirit proof containers are available. Although disposable syringes are for single use only most diabetics re-use syringes until the needle becomes too blunt to use (usually about 14 injections). After use air is drawn into the syringe

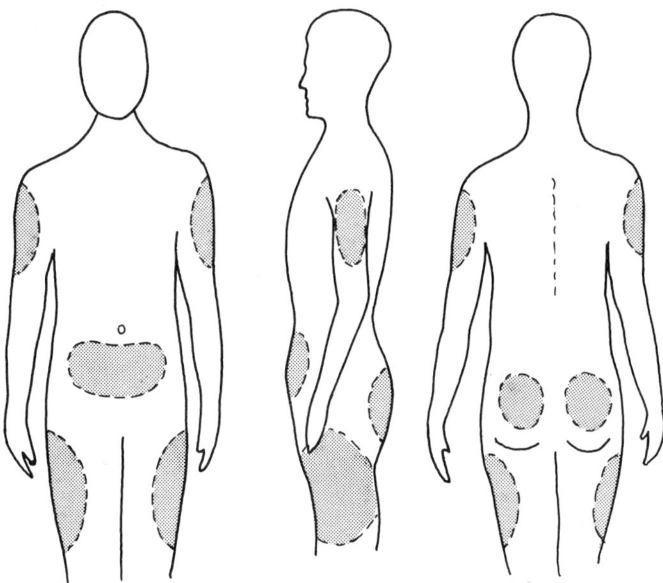

Figure 4.5 Insulin injection sites.

and expelled a few times to remove any residual insulin. The cap is then placed over the needle and the syringe is stored in a cool place ready for the next injection. No sterilization is necessary. This considerably reduces the burden of the ritual of insulin injections for the diabetic.

(b) Needles

If glass syringes are used then disposable needles $\frac{5}{8}''$ long 27/28 gauge should be used. Disposable needles may be used several times until they become blunt. Non-disposable needles are still used by some patients. These should be 27/28 gauge $\frac{5}{8}''$ long. It should go without saying that needles that are reused without sterilization should only be used by one person.

(c) Swabbing skin

In the past diabetics have been advised to swab the skin with spirit before the injection. It is now considered unnecessary to go through this ritual.

(d) Drawing up the insulin

It is important to teach patients to inject air into the insulin bottles before they attempt to draw insulin out. If they do not do this then they will create a vacuum in the insulin bottle and the withdrawal of insulin will be difficult. An attempt to suck insulin out of the bottle that contains a vacuum will result in air being drawn into the syringe and bubble errors created. When drawing up two types of insulin into a syringe for the twice daily regimen, it is important to draw up clear insulin first and then follow this with the cloudy insulin. When using this technique it is vital to inject air into the bottles first as failure to do so may result in insulin from the syringe being sucked back into the insulin bottle by the vacuum previously created. This will contaminate the longer acting insulin with the short-acting insulin and the bottle of insulin will then have to be thrown away.

(e) Sites for injection of insulin

Injections sites should be changed on a daily basis. The outer aspects of the thighs, the abdomen, and the arms should be used in turn (Figure 4.5). Repeated injection into one site should be avoided as this tends to produce fibrosis and fatty tumour development (Plate 3). This results in irregular absorption of the insulin and may be a cause of poor diabetic control. In children there is a tendency to do this as the sites that are repeatedly injected with insulin often become painless. It is important to remember that the rate of insulin absorption depends on the site of injection. Absorption from the leg is different from the arm or from the abdomen. Exercise will affect the rate of absorption. Only experience will tell the diabetic what to do.

(f) Injection technique

This may only be learned by practical demonstration. The skin should be stretched tight like a drum to allow rapid needle penetration and a painless injection. The needle should be inserted at near a right angle to the surface of the skin. The needle must go right through the skin into the subcutaneous tissues. Failure to do this will result in intradermal injection, poor absorption, and ulceration. After insertion of the needle the plunger should be gently withdrawn to test for intravenous placing of the needle. If no blood is withdrawn then the injection should be made.

4.7 HOME MONITORING

Monitoring the standard of control achieved in the home may be done by urine testing or blood glucose measurements.

4.7.1 Urine testing

The blood glucose concentration at which glucose appears in the urine will depend on the renal threshold for glucose (on average around 10 mmol/1 or 180 mg%). This renal threshold may increase with age and in renal disease. It must always be borne in mind, particularly when the urine tests do not correlate with blood glucose estimations. If the renal threshold for glucose is 10 mmol/1 then the blood glucose is twice normal before glucose appears in the urine. For good control the urine should be totally free of glucose.

4.7.2 Methods

There are now many methods for testing the urine for glucose. The old Clinitest tablet system has now been largely replaced by dip stix. Of these, those made by Ames (Diastix) and Bochringer (Diabur) are the most well known.

The basic rules for urine testing are set out below.

4.7.3 Non-insulin dependent diabetes

1. The urine should be tested in order to detect the postprandial glucose peaks.
2. The urine should be tested on rising first thing in the morning.
3. The bladder should be emptied before breakfast and the first urine specimen passed after breakfast should be tested.
4. The bladder should be emptied before the midday meal and the first urine specimen passed after the meal should be tested.
5. The bladder should be emptied before the evening meal and the first urine specimen passed after the evening meal should be tested.
6. Initially the urine should be tested four times per day. However, as soon as tests show no glycosuria testing may be reduced to once per day. It is important to rotate the tests throughout the day in the manner shown in *Table 4.4*. This will allow an assessment

Table 4.4 Urine tests for non-insulin treated diabetes

Date	*On waking*	*After breakfast*	*After midday meal*	*After evening meal*	*Notes*
3–11–86	0%				
4–11–86		$\frac{1}{4}$%			
5–11–86			2%		
6–11–86				1%	
7–11–86	0%				
8–11–86		$\frac{1}{2}$%			
9–11–86			2%		
				etc.	

of the degree of glycosuria, if any, not only throughout the weeks but also throughout the day.

4.7.4 Insulin treated diabetes

The aim in testing the urine in insulin treated diabetics is to detect glycosuria occurring preprandially.

The urine should be tested four times daily until good control is achieved. The frequency of testing may then be reduced to suit individual needs but should be at least one per day at varying times throughout the day.

Table 4.5 Urine/blood test for the insulin treated diabetic

Date	*Before breakfast*	*Before midday meal*	*Before evening meal*	*Before bedtime*	*Notes*
3–11–86	7.4				
4–11–86		9.2			
5–11–86			3.1		
6–11–86				5.4	
7–11–86	8.4				
8–11–86		10.4			
9–11–86			5.0		
10–11–86				6.0	
	etc.				

The aim is to assess the blood glucose level before each main meal. The bladder should be emptied and then 30 minutes later the bladder emptied again and this is the specimen that should be tested (post-voided urine test). It should be understood that this advice is easy to give to a patient but is not so easy for the patient to achieve.

The urine should be tested before breakfast, before the midday meal, before the evening meal, and before going to bed.

The results should be charted as in *Table 4.5*.

4.7.5 Home blood glucose monitoring (see also appendix 2)

There are now several systems in use for home blood glucose monitoring. Here the patient learns to prick the finger and with the resultant drop of blood estimate blood glucose concentrations by a colour change on a reagent strip. In the Ames Dextrostix system blood is left in contact with the reagent strip for one minute. It is then washed off and the resultant colour developed is read either against the scale given by the makers or in a meter. There are many meters on the market which will read the Ames Dextrostix. The disadvantage of this system is that the blood must be washed off from the strip. The Ames Glucostix and Visidex Stix, and also the test strips by BCL (Chemstrip BG, BM test Glycemie 20–800 R/1 – 44 Haemo-Glucotest 20–800) do away with the necessity for washing the blood off the stix. Here the blood is wiped off the strip with a tissue and again the colour developed read on a scale provided by the makers or in a meter. Again there are many meters on the market that will read the test strips.

Patients should be individually taught how to obtain blood from the fingers and how to apply it to the test strip. They should be taught how to use their own meters and how to avoid errors.

Probably the most common error is that of not getting enough blood on the test area. Hypodermic needles should not be used to prick the finger as these tend to produce a small deep hole which is painful but does not yield very much blood. It is better to use a lancet specifically designed for the purpose.

Swabbing the skin with alcohol may damage the enzymes on the test strip and is not necessary. It is preferable to wash the hands in warm water as this improves the perfusion of the skin and makes it easier to get the necessary amount of blood.

Accurate timing is important and in the case of Dextrostix the correct washing-off technique followed by blotting afterwards is essential.

Results should be recorded as in *Table 4.5*.

Information on test strips, meters, finger pricking devices, and lancets may be obtained from the various publications of the American and British Diabetic Association.

4.8 CONCLUSIONS

The potential benefits from maintaining normoglycaemia are immense. Successful treatment with insulin is a complex undertaking. Self-medication requires a high degree of knowledge, skill and motivation on the part of the patient. Education of a diabetic remains the corner-stone of successful practice.

FURTHER READING

British Diabetic Association Publications, 10 Queen Anne Street, London W1M 0BD.

Publications include:
The Diabetic Handbook – information on all topics related to diabetics.
Balance – A magazine published every 2 months for BDA members.
Countdown – A guide giving carbohydrate content of manufactured foods.
Better Cookery for Diabetics – A recipe book.
Cooking the New Diabetic Way – A high-fibre recipe book for the calorie conscious.

The Diabetics Diet Book – A new high fibre eating programme, Dr Jim Mann and the Oxford Dietetic Group. Martin Dunitz Positive Health Care Guide Series.

American Diabetes Association, 2 Park Avenue, New York, NY 10016
Professional Education Publications

Diabetes Care reprints:
Principles of nutrition and dietary recommendations for individuals with fructose, xylitol and sorbitol.
Fast food restaurants.
Measurement of blood glucose.
Counselling.
Glycaemic effects of carbohydrates.

Booklet:
A Guide for Professionals: The Effective Application of Exchange Lists for Meal Planning.

· Five ·

Diabetic emergencies

5.1 HYPOGLYCAEMIA

Hypoglycaemia is a common occurrence in patients treated with insulin. Its manifestations vary from a mild alteration in behaviour noticed only by relatives to severe hypoglycaemia resulting in death. Fortunately, considering the frequency of hypoglycaemia the latter is uncommon. In non-insulin treated diabetics hypoglycaemia may also occur in those patients treated with oral hypoglycaemic agents. This is usually due to inappropriate or incorrect use.

The incidence of hypoglycaemia may be increasing as diabetologists attempt to tighten diabetic control in order to prevent long-term complications. In the United States severe hypoglycaemia was reported in a series of patients being treated with continuous subcutaneous insulin infusion. There is, however, some evidence that small frequent doses of insulin with better diabetic control reduces the incidence of hypoglycaemia.

Even minor hypoglycaemia has important implications for the diabetic driver.

5.1.1 Causes

Hypoglycaemia is usually caused by one or a combination of the following three factors:

1. A late meal.
2. Unaccustomed or excessive exercise.
3. Mistakes in insulin dosage.

It will be seen that these factors are all under the control of the patient. The most important factor in the treatment and prevention of hypoglycaemia is patient education. Deliberate overdose with suicidal intent is not an uncommon cause of death due to hypoglycaemia.

5.1.2 Signs and symptoms

Hypoglycaemia produces signs and symptoms by adrenergic discharge and by neuroglycopenia. The onset may be slow with minor alterations in behaviour noticed only by relatives. At the other extreme the onset may be rapid leading to sudden unconsciousness without warning and followed by neuroglycopenic fits. Patients usually recognize the early symptoms of hypoglycaemia and are then able to take the appropriate evasive action. They may experience hunger, trembling, tingling sensations in the limbs and around the mouth. This is often associated with sweating. Early morning headaches may be a clue to nocturnal hypoglycaemia. All insulin-treated diabetics (except those with symptomatic coronary artery disease) should have a minor hypoglycaemic episode induced under controlled circumstances to allow them to recognize the early symptoms. In a doubtful situation home blood glucose monitoring is helpful in deciding whether the patient is hypoglycaemic. However, at the lower end of the scale (less than 3 mmol/1, 54 mg%) blood test strips are inaccurate and cannot be relied upon. If there is any doubt, the patient should take carbohydrate.

5.1.3 Differential diagnosis

The distinction between hyper- and hypoglycaemia is often a source of anxiety to medical students and newly qualified practitioners. However, the conditions are quite different and quite separate. In hypoglycaemia the patient has neuroglycopenic symptoms and symptoms of an adrenergic discharge. In hyperglycaemia the patient does not. The onset of hypoglycaemia is rapid whereas the onset of hyperglycaemia is gradual. In hyperglycaemia the patient is dehydrated and ketones may be present in the patient's breath. In hypoglycaemia the patient is not dehydrated.

There is usually no difficulty in differentiating between hyper- and hypoglycaemia. However, if there is any doubt intravenous glucose should be given. It can do no harm to the patient with hyperglycaemia but more insulin given to a patient in hypoglycaemic coma can be fatal.

5.1.4 Prevention and treatment

The most important factor in the treatment and prevention of hypoglycaemia is good patient education. Better diabetic control with multiple (twice daily or thrice daily) insulin injections will reduce the frequency of hypoglycaemia.

Patients must be taught to carry glucose with them and take this whenever symptoms first appear. They should be advised to take a meal before driving a motor vehicle and should never drive immediately before a meal particularly if there is likely to be any delay.

Relatives of patients particularly prone to hypoglycaemia (e.g. children) should be given a disposable glucagon pack and taught how to use it. This consists of a disposable syringe and a vial of glucagon (1 mg) which may be given intramuscularly or subcutaneously if the patient is not able to take carbohydrate by mouth. This often has a tremendous psychological effect on the family as a fail-safe mechanism. Just having it in the house boosts the morale of worried parents. It must be remembered that the shelf life of glucagon is 1 year and it must be replaced at yearly intervals.

Doctors should carry the following in their emergency kit:

1. Glucagon 1 mg in a disposable pack.
2. Dextrose solution 50% weight/volume (e.g. Minijet System, IMS 50 ml size).

As soon as a patient has recovered sufficient consciousness to take food by mouth he/she must be fed. If this is not done then the patient may lapse back into unconsciousness as the effects of emergency treatment wears off. This is particularly so with glugagon.

Patients requiring hospital treatment for hypoglycaemia represent a failure in patient education and in primary health care.

5.2 HYPERGLYCAEMIA

Hyperglycaemia may occur with or without ketoacidosis.

In a district general hospital serving a population of 250 000, 20–30 cases of hyperglycaemia with ketoacidosis may be seen each year. On the other hand, a doctor in primary health with a list of 2500 patients might expect to see only 1 case in 3–5 years.

5.2.1 Mortality

In a study of deaths in diabetics under the age of 50 years in the UK, delays in the diagnosis and treatment at both the primary and secondary health care level were found to be significant causes of mortality in hyperglycaemia with ketoacidosis. Even in good centres a mortality of 5–10% might be expected and in the average district general hospital it may be as high as 20–25%. In the elderly the mortality may rise to as much as 50%.

5.2.2 Pathogenesis

Severe insulin deficiency leads to hyperglycaemia secondary to hepatic gluconeogenesis and glycogenolysis. Uninhibited ketogenesis results in ketoacidosis. Intracellular acidosis produces a net transfer of intracellular potassium via the cell membrane to the extracellular space in order to maintain ionic equilibrium. With a rise in extracellular potassium concentrations severe potassium deficiency occurs owing to loss of potassium in the urine with the coincident osmotic diuresis. If the pH falls below 6.8 death is likely. Acidosis causes insulin resistance.

5.2.3 Precipitating factors

These may be listed as follows:

1. Intercurrent illness such as infection, myocardial infarction and cerebrovascular episodes.
2. A decrease in insulin dose on the mistaken advice of the doctor when the patient has some intercurrent illness.
3. Surgery and trauma.
4. A failure to take insulin.
5. Delayed diagnosis in a new diabetic.

It will be seen that prevention must lie in patient education and also in educating the primary health care worker. During any illness the patient must be encouraged to take a high fluid intake and increase the dose of insulin according to home blood glucose monitoring. However, if vomiting occurs and i.v. replacement therapy becomes necessary, admission should not be delayed.

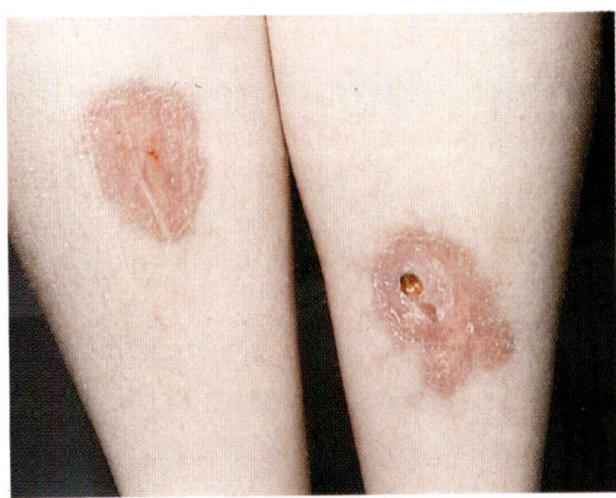

Plate 1 Necrobiosis lipoidica diabeticorum. Female aged 19 years, duration of non-insulin dependent diabetes 5 years.

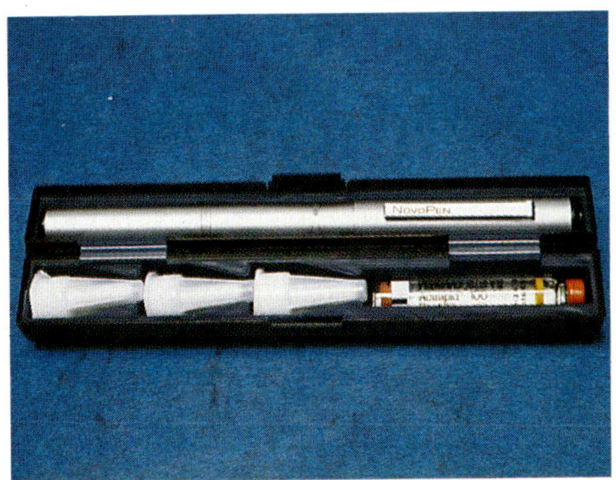

Plate 2 The Novopen.

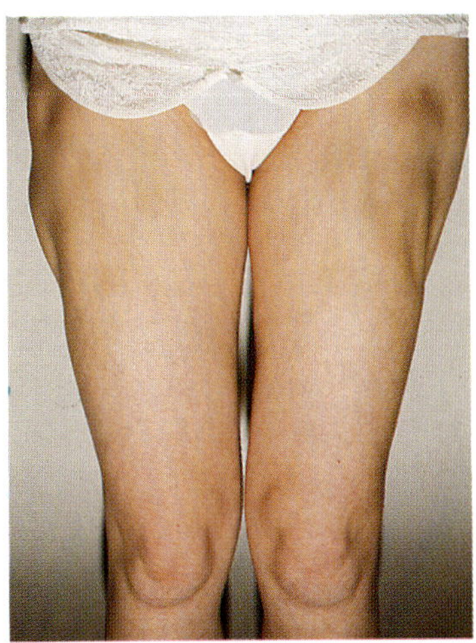

Plate 3 Fat atrophy. Miss S.A., aged 36, duration of diabetes 30 years. Fat atrophy associated with twice daily injections of Soluble and NPH insulin of beef origin.

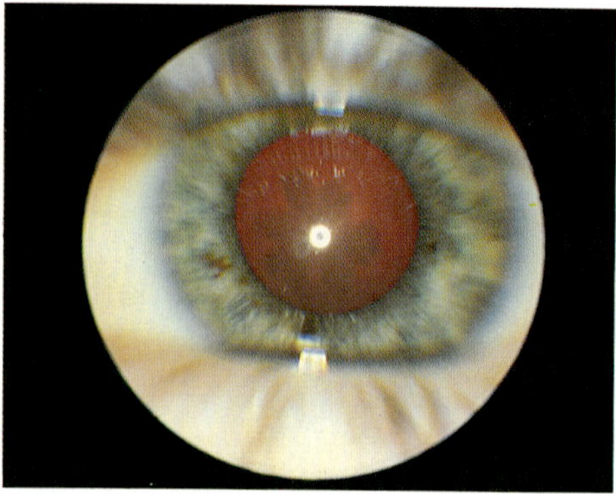

Plate 4 Snowflake cataract. Patient aged 20 years, newly diagnosed diabetes. Severe impairment of visual acuity. Visual acuity impairment appeared during presenting episode of severe ketoacidosis, resolved completely with normal visual acuity on recovery.

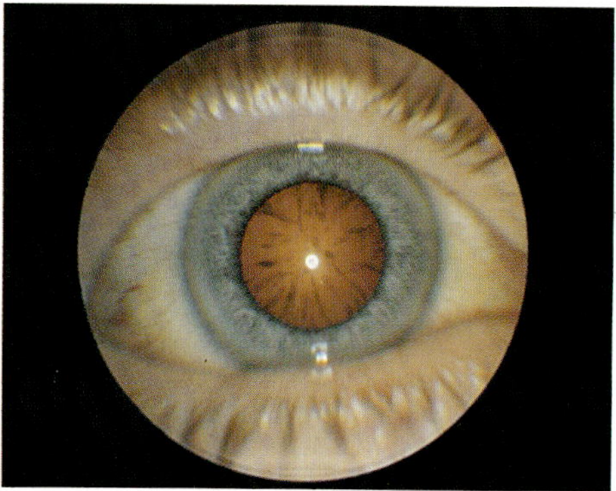

Plate 5 Senile cataract. Patient aged 65 years, duration of diabetes 10 years. The lens contains bar-like opacities which are described as having a roman numeral or cuneiform appearance and show up as black bars against the red reflex of the fundus. The central part of the lens may not be affected initially and visual acuity is thus preserved.

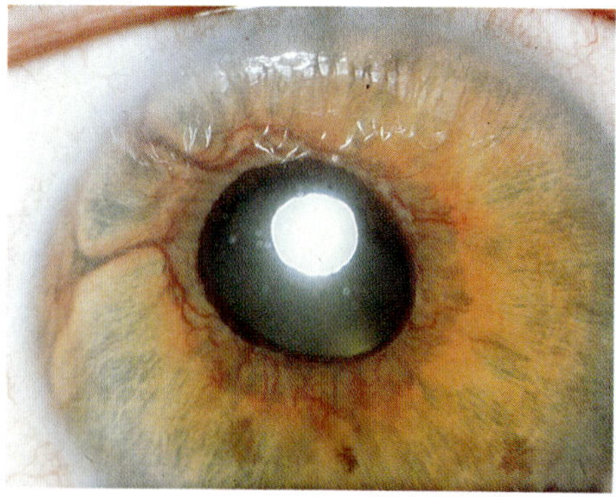

Plate 6 Rubeosis iridis with rubeotic glaucoma. (Reproduced with the kind permission of Mr. Peter Barry, FRCS, and the National Eye Institute (DRVS) Bethesda, USA.)

5.2.4 Presentation

Some patients with undiagnosed diabetes present with hyperglycaemic ketoacidotic precoma or coma. There is often a history of vague fatigue and weight loss. Direct questioning will usually reveal evidence of polyuria and polydipsia. The duration of the symptoms may be weeks or months. Intercurrent illness, particularly infection, may be the dominant feature and mask the underlying illness. Vomiting and abdominal pain may be mistaken for a surgical emergency. With progressive water and electrolyte imbalance severe leg cramps and abdominal pain mimicking the acute abdomen may be prominent. With progressive ketoacidosis breathlessness may be a prominent feature in the later stages.

5.2.5 Signs

Severe dehydration and ketoacidosis are mainly responsible for the signs. The skin is warm and dry. The skin loses its turgor, and (with increasing dehydration) the muscles have a texture of wet cardboard. Ocular tension is lost and if dehydration proceeds peripheral vascular shutdown will occur and the patient becomes shocked. Signs of shock include a cold cyanosed periphery, tachycardia, a loss of peripheral pulses, and a fall in blood pressure.

Hyperventilation (Kussmaul respiration) is a grave sign indicating severe ketoacidosis with increasing acidaemia. The patient smells strongly of ketones. Some doctors find this smell difficult to detect.

In contrast to hypoglycaemia higher cerebral functions are preserved at first. However, if the patient develops shock cerebral perfusion may be compromised and the patient develops precoma confusion and eventually deep coma.

Patients often have severe infections. However, only 10% of patients have a fever and mild hypothermia is not uncommon.

Early diagnosis is essential if the mortality is to be reduced. If the patient has sought medical advice and the diagnosis is delayed then the development of precoma or coma represents a major failure in primary health care. The patient must be admitted to a suitable unit without delay.

5.2.6 Initial investigations

In primary health care – blood glucose (finger prick, test strip). It is important to note that the accuracy of test strips depends on the skill and experience of the doctor or nurse. Urine (if available) test for acetone.

In secondary health care – in Accident and Emergency Department – i.e. before transfer to the ward:

1. Blood glucose.
2. Plasma urea.
3. Plasma electrolytes.
4. Full blood picture (haematocrit).
5. Blood pH (hydrogen ion concentration), pCO_2 and pO_2.
6. Blood ketones.
7. Catheter specimen of urine for microscopy, culture, ketones and sugar.
8. Blood culture
9. Throat swabs.
10. Chest X-ray.
11. ECG (the patient should remain connected to the monitor).

5.2.7 Treatment

As soon as the diagnosis is confirmed or even suspected with a high probability treatment should begin. The most important first aid treatment is rehydration. It is not simple lack of insulin that will kill the patient but dehydration. If there is to be any significant delay then rehydration should start with normal saline in primary health care.

5.2.8 Rehydration

Rehydration alone will lower the blood sugar and will considerably improve the patient's general state. The peripheral circulation will be restored and the urine flow re-established. If the patient is not vomiting then it may be possible to rehydrate the patient orally. However, intravenous rehydration is usually necessary. Peripheral veins may be used but a central line allows central venous manometry to be carried out in severely ill patients. This is particularly useful in the elderly and eliminates the risk of fluid overload.

Initial rehydration should begin with normal saline (containing 155 mmol/1 (milliequivalents per litre)). Excessive quantities of this solution will produce hypernatraemia. It may be necessary to use half-normal saline or even 5 or 10% dextrose. Half-normal saline or dextrose solution should replace normal saline when the serum sodium rises to 155 mmol/1 (155 mEq/1) or when blood glucose falls to less than 10 mmol/1 (180 mg%).

The rate of infusion will depend on the severity of the dehydration. *Table 5.1* may be used as a guide to the rate of infusion.

Table 5.1 Rehydration. Rate of i.v. infusion

Time (hours)	*Time interval (hours)*	*Volume of solution (litres)*	*Sodium (mmol)*
0–1	1	2	310
1–2	1	1	155
2–3	1	1	155

I.V. infusion should be continued until the central venous pressure is normal, the patient is fully rehydrated, peripheral perfusion has been restored, and the patient has stopped vomiting and can take oral fluids. On average 4–6 litres of fluid are retained in the first 48 hours indicating the size of deficit at onset.

5.2.9 Treatment with insulin

Low dose insulin regimens have now become standard practice in the treatment of diabetic ketoacidosis. Two regimens are at present used. The low-dose intramuscular regimen of Alberti is particularly useful if high-quality nursing supervision is not available. The low-dose insulin intravenous infusion regimen of Sonksen is very effective and easily controlled when the patient can be admitted to an intensive therapy unit.

5.2.10 Low-dose intramuscular regimen

In this regimen insulin is given intramuscularly and it is therefore essential that adequate rehydration be achieved before insulin is given otherwise the insulin will not be absorbed.

Neutral Soluble (Regular) or Human Actrapid insulin is used. The low dose intramuscular regimen is shown in *Table 5.2*.

Table 5.2 Low-dose intramuscular regimen

Time (hours)	*Dose (units of insulin)*
0	20
1	6
2	6
3	6

This regimen is followed until the blood glucose has fallen to 10 mmol/1 (180 mg%). Five units of insulin are then given every 2 hours to maintain a steady blood glucose of around 10 mmol/1 (180 mg%).

If blood glucose levels do not fall in the first 2 hours it is essential to give insulin intravenously.

5.2.11 Low-dose intravenous infusion

It is important to realize that the plasma half life of insulin is only 4 minutes. Should the insulin infusion be stopped or the i.v. line become disconnected the patient will have no effective insulin circulating within 4 minutes. This is the reason for the prerequisite of good nursing care with constant monitoring in an intensive therapy unit.

Neutral Soluble (regular) insulin or Human Actrapid insulin should be used. It should be given by an intravenous line preferably separate from other venous lines although it may be piggy backed on to a central venous line.

The insulin is best administered by a separate syringe pump. However, it is also possible to mix the insulin in the infusion solution if a pump is not available.

Insulin should be infused at a rate of 4–6 units per hour until the blood glucose is 10 mmol/1 (180 mg%) and then 1–0.5 units per hour to maintain a steady blood glucose of around 7–10 mmol/1 (125–180 mg%).

5.2.12 Correction of electrolyte imbalance

(a) Sodium and chloride

Sodium and chloride replacement is adequately taken care of by the rehydration regimen indicated above.

(b) Potassium

Initial serum potassium measurements may be high. As indicated earlier intracellular acidosis produces a net transfer of intracellular potassium to the extracellular space. The high serum potassium may lull the doctor into a false sense of security. Despite the high serum potassium there is usually a severe total body deficit of potassium. As soon as rehydration starts and insulin is given plasma potassium concentration falls dramatically. Severe hypokalaemia may result and may be responsible for the patient's death when all appears to be going well. Potassium should therefore be given early in the rehydration process and the level of plasma potassium monitored throughout.

Potassium should be replaced by mixing potassium chloride in the normal saline solution used to rehydrate the patient. *Table 5.3* indicates a suitable dosage schedule for potassium.

Table 5.3 Potassium replacement

Plasma potassium concentration (mmol/l)	*Dose (mmol/hr)*
Greater than 5	0
4–5	13
3–4	26
Less than 3	39

5.2.13 Correction of acid base deficit

Appropriate rehydration and insulin therapy usually suffices to correct the acid base deficit. However, if the blood pH is less than 7, insulin resistance becomes a problem and life is threatened. If the pH is 7 or less then bicarbonate solution should be given. This will accentuate hypokalaemia and it is essential to give extra potassium.

Aliquots of 50 ml 8.4% sodium bicarbonate solution together with 13 mmol of added potassium should be given over a 20 minute period. After an equilibration period of approximately 10 minutes the pH should be estimated again. The process should be repeated until the pH is greater than 7. However, it is important to realize that for evey mmol of bicarbonate given 1 mmol of sodium will also be given. This may result in a life-threatening hypernatraemia. The resulting hyperosmolarity will produce intracellular dehydration and a prolongation of coma. Under no circumstances should infusions containing 250–500 ml 8.4% sodium bicarbonate solutions be set up as there is a real danger that these may be run in accidentally and kill the patient.

It is worth noting that as little as 50 ml bicarbonate will relieve the distressing hyperventilation due to ketoacidosis.

5.2.14 Practical points in the management of diabetic ketoacidosis

1. Blood glucose should be monitored at the bedside using blood glucose test strips and a meter. Initially blood glucose should be measured every 30 minutes and values should be checked by the laboratory every 4 hours. It is important not to leave this task to an inexperienced nurse.

   Inaccurate information is more dangerous than no information at all.
2. Insulin may adhere to giving sets and syringes. This may lower the actual quantity of insulin infused. It has been suggested that human serum albumin, polygeline, plasma protein fractions or 2 mls of the patient's own blood should be added to infusions containing insulin. This binds the insulin and prevents it sticking to equipment. It has been my own personal experience that this is unnecessary.
3. If blood levels do not fall within the first hour the rate of insulin infusion should be doubled after checking that the pump is still working and connected to patient!
4. Switched off intravenous insulin pumps or disconnected insulin pumps are the commonest cause of failure of the low-dose i.v. insulin regimen!
5. Even if the plasma potassium is greater than 5 mmol/1 on initial investigation, with rehydration and insulin therapy the potassium may drop dramatically in the first hour and must be monitored.
6. Although ECG monitoring is sometimes helpful, the plasma potassium may be less than 2 mmol/1 before definite ECG signs occur and this is too late. Tented T waves suggest hyperkalaemia and flat T waves with T wave inversion indicate hypokalaemia.

7. Patients with ketoacidosis may develop gastric dilatation. The stomach can sequestrate several litres of electrolyte-rich fluid and a nasogastric tube should be passed in patients with ketoacidosis developing precoma or coma to prevent vomiting and the danger of aspiration pneumonia.
8. Antibiotic cover should be given in all cases since most patients with ketoacidosis either have an infection or are liable to severe infection.
9. Patients with severe dehydration or a hyperosmolar state should be heparinized to prevent localized thromboses and diffuse intravascular coagulation syndrome.
10. If the patient remains oliguric or anuric after adequate rehydration with a central venous pressure greater than 1 cm and a systolic blood pressure greater than 100 mm Hg, then Frusemide 120 mg i.v. should be given. If this fails the patient should be treated as having acute renal failure.
11. If the systolic blood pressure fails to rise above 80 mm Hg despite adequate rehydration, 2 units of whole blood should be given.
12. If the pO_2 is less than 11 kPa (80 mm Hg) oxygen via a face mask or a nasal catheter should be given.

5.2.15 Hyperglycaemia without ketoacidosis leading to pre-coma or coma

5–10% of patients having hyperglycaemia leading to precoma or coma do not have ketoacidosis. These patients are usually elderly and non-insulin dependent diabetics. This condition is sometimes associated with severe polydipsia and polyuria treated by an excessive intake of sweetened drinks. Patients with hyperglycaemia without significant ketoacidosis probably have enough circulating insulin to switch off ketogenesis but not enough to prevent the rapid rise in blood glucose concentration. Blood glucose concentrations in excess of 50 mmol/1 are seen. In this hyperosmolar state dehydration is the most significant sign. An osmolarity greater than 360 mmol/1 is usual. The signs and symptoms are similar to those of hyperglycaemia with ketoacidosis without symptoms relating to the acidosis.

(a) Treatment

This is essentially similar to the treatment of hyperglycaemia with ketoacidosis. However, rehydration is even more urgent. The danger of contributing to the osmotic imbalance cannot be overemphasized. If the plasma sodium is 150 mmol/1 or more then half-normal saline or 5% dextrose should be used in place of normal saline. A central venous line is desirable.

Fortunately, these patients are usually sensitive to even small doses of insulin and lowering the blood glucose concentration is usually not difficult.

The risk of diffuse intravascular coagulation and post coma venous thrombosis is very high in these patients. Heparin should be used prophylactically.

In patients with prolonged severe dehydration, anuria with uraemic acidosis or lacticacidosis may follow. These patients may need treatment with peritoneal dialysis.

5.3 DIABETES AND SURGERY

There is no doubt that good metabolic control in the pre, peri- and post-operative periods of surgery have important effects. Normoglycaemia reduces the length and severity of the post-operative catabolic state. It reduces the danger of infection and increases the rate of wound healing.

Anaesthetists often fear hypoglycaemia during surgery. Good metabolic control may be achieved and the anaesthetist's task made easier by adherence to the following simple rules:

1. Blood glucose should be monitored before, during and after surgery. Test strips and a meter are quite adequate.
2. Particularly in cold cases, pre-operative blood glucose values should be between 3 and 7 mmol/1.
3. For the diabetic controlled by diet alone there is usually no problem pre-operatively. The patient should be treated as if a non diabetic on the day of operation. However, post-operatively blood glucose should be monitored closely as there is often a post-operative rise in blood glucose due to the stress of the surgery.
4. For diabetics controlled on oral hypoglycaemic agents together

with a diet, the patient should be fasted pre-operatively in the usual way and not be given an oral hypoglycaemic agent on the day of operation. As Chlorpropamide is a long acting oral hypoglycaemic agent it should be stopped at least 24 hours before operation.

5. For insulin treated diabetics undergoing minor surgery it may only be necessary to fast the patient and not give the insulin on the morning of the operation. This presupposes of course, that the patient is first on the list and first thing in the morning. It is also important to remember that a longer acting insulin given the night before operation e.g. Monotard, may still be acting in the morning and not covered by carbohydrate because the patient has been fasted. A reduction in the evening dose of Monotard on the night before the operation will prevent this problem occurring. Again simple monitoring of blood glucose values before, during and after the operation is essential. After minor procedures the patient may be fed immediately and then given short acting insulins to cover the carbohydrate intake. On the day following the procedure the patient should return to his normal diet and normal insulin regimen.
6. For all insulin-treated diabetics undergoing major surgery and for any other diabetic who is poorly controlled pre-operatively the following regimen is recommended. The regimen is called the PIG regimen from the contents of the i.v. infusion (Potassium, Insulin and Glucose).

For 3 days pre-operatively the patient should be stabilized on a twice or thrice daily insulin regimen. A short-acting insulin such as Soluble or Actrapid should be given with each main carbohydrate intake and Monotard or Isophane insulin should be given in the evening to control blood glucose levels through the night.

On the day of operation an intravenous infusion should be set up. This should consist of 10% dextrose, 500 ml Actrapid Insulin 10 units, potassium chloride 1 g.

500 ml of this solution should be infused over a 4–5 hour period and be continued until oral feeding restarts. Blood glucose and potassium concentration should be estimated at frequent intervals and the rate of insulin infusion and the amount of potassium added to the infusion should be varied accordingly. A guide to this adjustment is shown in *Table 5.4*.

Table 5.4 Potassium–insulin–glucose infusion

Blood glucose results	*Insulin dose*
Up to 5 mmol/l	5 units/500 ml 10% dextrose
5–9 mmol/l	10 units/500 ml 10% dextrose
10–19 mmol/l	15 units/500 ml 10% dextrose
Greater than 20 mmol/l	20 units/500 ml 10% dextrose
Plasma potassium (mmol/l)	*Potassium infusion rate* (mmol/hr)
Greater than 5	0
4–5	13
3–4	26
Less than 3	39

The PIG regimen indicated above may be varied by using a low-dose insulin infusion pump. Here the dextrose and potassium are given by one line and the insulin is administered by a separate infusion pump at a rate of 2–5 units per hour. This allows tighter control of the blood glucose but requires a higher standard of nursing care. With the straight PIG regimen when glucose is given the insulin is given concomitantly. However, when using a separate infusion pump the patient may receive an infusion of insulin and the dextrose infusion may be inadvertently turned off or reduced.

Insulin and glucose should be administered by a separate i.v. line from that used for other infusions such as saline and blood since it is often necessary during surgical procedures to increase the rate of infusion of blood and saline.

It is also important to remember that the stresses associated with a surgical procedure and an anaesthetic coupled with i.v. glucose infusions may cause severe hyperglycaemia even in patients normally very well controlled on diet alone, or diet with an oral hypoglycaemic agent. It follows that blood glucose must be monitored if good metabolic control is to be maintained.

In the post-operative period normoglycaemia should be the aim. In patients receiving i.v. infusions of insulin the infusion rates should be adjusted to maintain blood glucose values between 3 and 7 mmol/1. When the patient returns to normal oral feeding then three doses of a short acting insulin should be given with each main carbohydrate intake and a single dose of Monotard or NPH given in the evening to control the nocturnal blood glucose levels.

As soon as would healing has been achieved and stitches have been removed the patient should be returned to his former diet and insulin regime. However, the stresses of surgery often remain for some time after operation and it is usually necessary to increase the pre-operative dose of insulin by about 20%. An additional 20% may be needed in the presence of infection or if steroids have been given.

5.4 DIABETES MELLITUS AND INTERCURRENT ILLNESS

Many patients and not a few doctors find it difficult to understand why blood glucose concentrations rise even when the patient is fasting. This is usually because they do not understand that the liver contributes significantly to blood glucose levels by hepatic gluconeogenesis and glycogenolysis. The hepatic contribution to blood glucose levels is enhanced by relative insulin deficiency, catecholamines, glucagon and cortisol. All these factors operate during illness. It therefore follows that even if the patient cannot eat during an illness, severe hyperglycaemia may result. The patient must receive his normal injection of insulin and if necessary this should be increased to control the blood glucose concentrations. Here the value of home blood glucose monitoring is evident. Patients should be encouraged to adjust their own insulin and give mutiple injections of short acting insulins (three or four times per day) to control blood glucose levels. This may save an unnecessary admission to hospital with diabetic ketoacidosis.

If the patient is not able to take a normal diet then he should be encouraged to take fluids containing carbohydrate. The following examples contain 20 g carbohydrate (2 standard portions):

1. A glass of milk containing 2 teaspoonfuls of Ovaltine, Horlicks or Bournvita.
2. 100 ml of fresh or tinned unsweetened orange juice containing 2 teaspoonfuls of sugar.
3. Diabetic fruit squash or lemon juice containing four teaspoonfuls of sugar.

See also section 4.4.

If the patient is vomiting or unable to take fluids then hyperglycaemia and ketoacidosis may develop rapidly. Patients not able to maintain oral hydration should be admitted to hospital without delay.

· Six ·

Diabetic follow-up

6.1 INTRODUCTION

The shorter Oxford English Dictionary defines follow-up as a continuation of action. At this point it is worth while reiterating the aims of treating diabetes (*see section 4.2*). The aim is to achieve a fit and happy patient leading a normal or near normal life style, with a normal or near normal blood glucose concentration without significant hypoglycaemia. By so doing it is hoped to prevent or delay long-term complications. We know that patients not being regularly followed up have a greater risk of early mortality (Deckert, 1978) and those patients who default from regular follow-up clinics often have poor glycaemic control and more retinopathy (Hammersley *et al.*, 1985). Having discovered diabetes, educated the diabetic to enable him to look after his or her own disease, treated the diabetes and attained the therapeutic and glycaemic goals, it is then necessary to organize life long follow-up to help the diabetic manage his chronic disease. The aims of follow-up are as follows:

1. To maintain patient morale.
2. To maintain patient's determination to continue self-care.
3. To continue education and revision.
4. To monitor glycaemic control (interval blood sugar/HbA1/ home blood glucose monitoring etc.).
5. To monitor weight.
6. To detect long-term complications at an early stage.
7. Advise on treatment.
8. To arrange an appointment and recall system.

The patient needs someone to whom he or she can turn in order to gain advice and support. It is important that a follow-up appointment should be regarded as part of boosting the patient's morale and fortifying his determination to continue self-care. To this end education and revision must continue. There must be regular monitoring of such parameters as glycaemic control, weight, blood pressure and a screening programme for the early detection of the long-term complications of diabetes. During follow-up further advice and treatment must be given. At the end of any follow-up interview it is essential to give a further appointment and to have some means of being sure that the patient keeps that appointment in order to maintain continuity of care. On the whole primary health care is demand led. This means that either treatment or advice or both are given on demand from the patient. The system is not geared up for anticipatory or preventative medicine. This is in contradistinction to secondary health care which has a formalized follow-up system in its outpatient departments. If primary health care is to take part in routine follow-up then a change in attitude and organization is necessary.

The attributes of a successful follow-up system are as follows:

1. An appointment and recall system.
2. Structured interviews at properly organized clinic sessions.
3. Documentation.
4. Audit.

It is important to have an appointment and recall system. Patients should be seen at organized clinic sessions with properly structured interviews. Clear documentation is essential if long-term trends are to be appreciated and audit carried out.

6.2 APPOINTMENT AND RECALL

In secondary health care there is an organized appointment system. Patients are given an appointment and they are expected to attend. If they do not there is a clear indication that they have not attended and a further appointment can be given. This of course is in theory. In many busy clinics in the UK if patients do not attend, there is a sigh of relief, and the patient is quietly forgotten! Non-attendance rates may be an indication that patients are voting with their feet, refusing to attend if they do not get a reasonable service or have to wait too long for it. However, there is no excuse in secondary health care for not chasing up non attenders and at least informing the primary health care physician that the patient has failed to keep an appointment.

In primary health care, as indicated above, the situation is quite different. It is necessary to organize *de novo* an appointment and recall system. Many practices in the United Kingdom now have appointment systems but often do not have recall systems. A practice age, sex, disease register, is a useful start to finding those patients who are at risk. Computerized systems are now available for appointments and for the recall of at-risk patients. However, a simple card index system may be all that is necessary to ensure that patients are regularly followed up and that if they do not attend they are given a further appointment (McCormack, 1976).

There are a number of diabetic patients who consistently fail to attend either clinic or the family doctor for follow-up. These patients are at risk from increased mortality and morbidity. The sanction of 'no follow-up – no supplies' should be applied.

6.3 THE STRUCTURED FOLLOW-UP INTERVIEW

No matter whether follow-up takes place in primary or secondary health care, the principles of follow-up are the same. The follow-up appointment should be divided into two halves: a nurse-conducted interview and a doctor-conducted interview.

6.3.1 Nurse-conducted interview

The nurse-conducted interview is structured as follows:

1. Weight.
2. Urine for glucose/albumin/acetone, urine to laboratory (MSU for culture if protein present, early morning urine for albumin/creatinine ratio in clinics monitoring early diabetic nephropathy (see Chapter 8).
3. Blood pressure – either sitting blood pressure, or lying and standing blood pressures.
4. Distant visual acuity followed by dilatation of the pupils if examination of the eyes is intended.
5. Removal of the shoes and socks with examination of the feet.
6. The organization of laboratory investigations preferably to provide a haemoglobin A1 and interval blood sugar for the

doctor on the day of interview. The serum creatinine and blood lipids measured on an annual basis.
7. Documentation – patient record card and clinic/practice record sheet.

Before the patient is seen by the doctor the nurse should weigh the patient, test an early morning urine sample for glucose, protein and acetone, measure blood pressure, test the distant visual acuity, and if necessary dilate the pupils. The shoes and socks should be removed and the feet examined. The results of previous investigations should be obtained. The results should be entered into the patient's record card and in the clinic or practice record sheet. The patient is then ready to be seen by the doctor.

6.3.2 Doctor conducted interview

The doctor-conducted interview is structured as follows:

1. Any problems?
2. Systematic enquiry – eyes, feet, neuropathy symptoms, chest pain, hypoglycaemia.
3. A review of home monitoring (home blood glucose or urine tests).
4. A review of laboratory results.
5. A review of nurse conducted interview results.
6. Clinical examination and organization of relevant investigations indicated.
7. Discuss with patient the standard of control achieved.
8. Review and change treatment if necessary. Record data in patient's record card and clinic/practice record sheet.
9. Arrange further follow-up appointment.

The interview should always begin with asking the patient whether there are 'any problems'. Having given the patient the opportunity of speaking first the doctor may then go on to ask specific questions relating to eyes, feet, neuropathy, and where appropriate chest pain. It is important to ask about hypoglycaemia. On the whole hypoglycaemia is under-reported by patients and may be over reported by relatives. A simple grading of hypoglycaemia is useful in documentation. A grade I hypoglycaemic episode involves the patient being aware of hypoglycaemia and taking corrective action without difficulty. A grade II hypoglycaemic episode necessitates the intervention of another person to give carbohydrate by mouth. A grade III hypoglycaemic episode requires treatment by a doctor either on a domiciliary visit or in an accident and emergency department. The timing of hypoglycaemia is crucial to the adjustment of treatment. It also has important medicolegal aspects which necessitate accurate recording in the notes.

The doctor should then review the patient's home monitoring whether it be by urine testing or blood glucose testing. These results should be compared with laboratory monitoring (interval blood sugar and HbA1). The information from the nurse-conducted interview should be reviewed.

The doctor should then make any examination and arrange any investigation he considers necessary.

After examination the standard of control achieved and the findings of the examination should be discussed. Any necessary changes in treatment should be made and a further follow-up appointment should be arranged.

A suggested follow-up interval for examination and investigation is as follows:

1. Follow-up interval 3–6 months.
2. Weight, urinary protein, acetone and glucose, interval blood sugar and HbA1. Interval 3–6 months.
3. Examination of the feet (particularly in the elderly), interval 3–6 months.
4. Examination for neuropathy and peripheral vascular disease. Interval 3–6 months.
5. Blood pressure measurement yearly or when indicated.
6. Distant visual acuity and fundoscopy. Retinopathy present, 3–6 months; retinopathy absent, yearly.
7. Inspection of injection sites in insulin treated diabetics – interval 6 months.
8. MSU if protein present – when indicated.
9. Early morning urine for albumin/creatinine ratio (to detect early nephropathy), 6 monthly in selected patients (see Chapter 8).

6.4 DOCUMENTATION

The problem of adequate documentation for the diabetic is a perennial one. Diabetes is a lifelong disease. The patient may live for 50 years or more. Each patient will have a large amount of data. There are a large number of patients. Anyone who has worked in a diabetic clinic will be only too familiar with the problem of being confronted with large, untidy, chaotic and unmanageable case notes. Vital sequential time-related data detailing the standard of control often cannot be found. In primary health care in the UK the situation is even worse. The Lloyd George case folder which was introduced in the 1920s has changed little. It is totally inadequate for the follow-up of chronic disease. Some doctors have introduced special case notes for diabetes (Tasker, 1984) using an A4 size folder and co-operation card.

In addition to doctor held primary and secondary health care notes the patient should have some form of co-operation card/co-operation book in which his results are recorded. *Table 6.1* shows the clinical record pages of the Poole Co-operation Record Book for diabetic patients. The vertical columns represent date, weight, interval blood sugar, HbA1, urine tests for sugar, protein and acetone, a check list for eyes, nervous system, cardiovascular system and feet, columns for diet (grams carbohydrate per day), insulin treatment, and oral hypoglycaemic therapy. A clear indication of the next visit is a helpful reminder for the patient. A check list is completed by simply ticking the relevant column when the system has been examined. The horizontal section labelled 'goals' enables the clinician to write in realistic goals for the patient to compare with results actually achieved. Clinical details of examination, e.g. visual acuity, fundoscopy, vibration sense, blood pressure etc. should be recorded in primary or secondary health care notes.

Whatever the method of recording information, it should be simple otherwise the records will not be kept. It is also important to have some form of cumulative sequential recording of numerical data in order that trends may be easily appreciated.

The computer may come to the rescue of those attempting to rationalize the mass of diabetic clinic notes (Hill, 1984, 1986).

6.5 FOLLOW-UP – WHERE?

In a non-organized diabetic system it is likely that at least 50% of all diabetics are neither attending the hospital diabetic clinic nor receiving regular care from their family doctor (Yudkin *et al.*, 1980). There are 30 health care districts in the United Kingdom which have no

Table 6.1 Clinical record
(Co-operation Record Book for Diabetic Patients)

		Blood tests		*Urine*			*Check-list*				*Diet*	*Insulin–units*					*Next*
Date	*Wt*	*IBS*	*HbA1*	G	*P*	*A*	*Eyes*	*NS*	*CVS*	*Feet*	G.CHO	*Type*	*AM*	*MD*	*PM*	*OHA*	*visit*
Goal		3–7	<8.5	0	0	0	*	*	*	*		—	—	—	—	—	—

diabetologist or organized diabetic service (Royal College of Physicians and British Diabetic Association Report, 1984). Even in a large centre with a recognized diabetologist the diabetic clinic may perform badly (Yudkin *et al.*, 1980). Only 75% of patients had either their eyes or blood pressure measured in the preceding 2 years of a survey, and less than 60% of patients had their feet examined. The performance figures will probably be worse for primary health care, the ordinary run of the mill diabetic clinic and for patients being followed-up in routine medical outpatients where no diabetic clinic is available. There is therefore considerable room for improvement and certainly a need for a rationalization of care. By organization it is possible to improve the standard of diabetic care within primary health care.

In Wolverhampton one third of the practices in the district have 'mini clinics'. These clinics are run by family doctors with a special interest in diabetes and look after 87% of all diabetics in the participating practices. Interestingly, the default rate from these clinics is only 6% compared with that of 31% of the hospital clinic (Singh *et al.*, 1984).

In the Community Care Service for Diabetics in the Poole Area, 37% of known patients are followed up in hospital and 63% of the patients are followed up by family doctors.

At this point it is worth while stressing the dangers of discharging patients from a diabetic clinic to primary health care without consultation and organization. In one series 14% of patients were not seen at all in primary health care and 20% thought that they were 'cured' (Wilkes and Laughton, 1980). In another study, follow-up in primary health care at 5 years had dropped to only 14% of the follow-up population (compared with 100% follow-up in the matched hospital population). In only 5% of the primary health care population had blood glucose been measured, and haemoglobin A1 levels were significantly higher. What was more disturbing, the mortality in the population followed up by the family doctors was three times that of the hospital population (Hayes and Harries, 1984).

However, all is not doom and gloom with regard to shared care. Both the Wolverhampton and the Poole studies show that with organization excellent control and follow-up can be achieved in primary health care.

There thus appears to be a wide spectrum in the nature of diabetic follow-up. A totally diabetic clinic orientated service almost certainly misses at least 50% of the diabetics in the district. Shared care may be limited as in the mini clinic system of Wolverhampton, or complete as in the Community Care Scheme for Diabetics in the Poole Area. At the other end of the spectrum total diabetic care may be undertaken by suitably interested and qualified family doctors with little or no participation of secondary health care (Tasker, 1984). This type of primary health care is excellent for isolated rural communities with no easy access to secondary health care.

A practitioner with a list of 2500 patients might expect to find 25 patients with diabetes. This would of course depend on the age structure of his practice. Within this group there would be 16 non-insulin dependent diabetics, and 9 insulin dependent diabetics. If we regard 30 patients as a reasonable number and assume that they are followed up twice yearly, then 60 appointments per annum will be needed. Allowing 20 minutes per patient this would require 20 hours per annum consultation time. Allowing for a 10-month year it would be necessary for such a practitioner to devote a 2 hour session to diabetes each month. Organization of ancillary service in primary health care is just as important as in secondary health care. In the United Kingdom two ancillary staff are allowed per principal GP with 70% of the costs being piad for by the family practitioner committee. The remaining 30% is tax deductable. Without such ancillary help it is unlikely that a doctor in primary health care would be able to undertake routine follow-up of even part of his diabetic population.

6.6 THE PROS AND CONS

From the patient's point of view routine follow-up by the family doctor has been found to be acceptable (Upton, 1975). Visiting the local family doctor's surgery (office) instead of the diabetic clinic usually involves far less travelling time and is therefore less expensive. The waiting time and time off work is greatly reduced and continuity of care is achieved because the patient sees one permanent family doctor.

From the family doctor's point of view it must be admitted that diabetic follow up does involve more work and does involve an increase in expenditure. However, the increased work load is not as great as one might expect from the above calculation and the slight increase in both work load and expenditure do not seem to deter the interested and motivated practitioner. It has been said that job satisfaction is increased and that by regular follow-up problems may be anticipated, prevented or treated before a situation becomes critical. (Russell *et al.*, 1974; Thorne and Russell, 1973). The overall work load may be decreased by preventative or anticipatory medicine although this is difficult to prove. Diabetes mellitus is a multisystem disease affecting the whole patient. By being clinically involved with the patient, the general practitioner may use the disease as a hone on which to sharpen his clinical ability, and gain individual job satisfaction.

From the secondary health care point of view, shared care provides the opportunity for an improvement of services to both patient and family doctor. The improved working conditions of the diabetologist with increased room to manoeuvre stimulates innovation and the development of the service.

The happy co-operation between the patient, primary health care, and secondary health care, increases the awareness of diabetes and its problems and in general boosts health service morale.

6.7 THE NEED FOR AUDIT

In any system of care an assessment of the standards achieved is essential. How else are we to assess our success? Comparisons need to be made and differences found need to be analysed. The subject is given fuller treatment in Chapter 14. The difficulty in collecting data from primary health care must not be underestimated. Any increase in the documentation required would significantly increase the work load and be a positive disincentive to family doctor participation in follow-up.

6.8 FOLLOW-UP IN PREGNANCY

6.8.1 The effect of pregnancy on diabetes

Pregnancy in the diabetic may upset metabolic control. Initially there is a decrease in insulin requirement (during the first 3 months) but later insulin requirement gradually increases. Immediately after the delivery there is a precipitous fall in insulin requirement and the patient may become hypoglycaemic.

Patients with long-term complications respond variably to pregnancy. Diabetic retinopathy may be unaltered, may even get better, but may dramatically get worse. In view of this patients should have their eyes examined at monthly intervals throughout the pregnancy. Pregnancy is not a contraindication to treatment with photocoagulation should the need arise. Diabetic nephropathy may worsen considerably during pregnancy.

6.8.2 The effects of diabetes on pregnancy

Diabetics are often subfertile and may have some considerable difficulty in conceiving (see section 6.8.3. (a)). Having conceived, abortions and miscarriages are more common.

The non-diabetic perinatal mortality rate is around 0.6% In one centre the diabetic mortality was 22.1% in 1946. Over the following 34 years the perinatal mortality rate was reduced to 4.4% by improved diabetic and obstetric management (Pedersen, 1977). The perinatal mortality increases as the age of onset of diabetes in the mother decreases. Similarly the perinatal mortality rate increases as the duration of diabetes mellitus increases. The presence of microvascular disease increases the perinatal mortality greatly (White, 1965).

Fifty per cent of the perinatal mortality in the children of diabetic mothers is caused by congenital malformations. The overall malformation rate in diabetics is 7.6% compared with 2.6% in non-diabetics. The fatal malformation rate is 2.7% in the children of diabetics compared with 0.4% in the children of non-diabetics.

It has been suggested that hyperglycaemia or its metabolic consequences is teratogenic. In a preconception clinic where good glycaemic control was achieved before conception, the major congenital abnormality rate was 5.6%. Without such preconception and periconception control the major congenital abnormality rate rose to 12.2% (Ylinen *et al.*, 1984).

6.8.3 Summary

1. Insulin requirement. Initially decreased. Later increased.
2. Variable effect on retinopathy and nephropathy.
3. Subfertility.
4. Higher risk of early abortion or miscarriage.
5. Increased perinatal mortality.
6. Increased incidence of congenital malformation.

6.8.4 Management of the diabetic during pregnancy

(a) Preconception management

Education must contain advice to would-be diabetic mothers. They should be encouraged to maintain good glycaemic control and should not smoke. They should seek advice on contraception. In the absence of other contraindications there is no specific diabetic contraindication to the contraceptive pill. However, in keeping with non-diabetics, diabetics on the contraceptive pill will gain weight and will in addition require an increased dose of insulin. The use of intrauterine devices is unsatisfactory and the rate of failure is higher in diabetics. If there are contraindications to the contraceptive pill then other forms of contraception should be discussed. This advice does not differ from that given to the non-diabetic.

The problems of subfertility should be explained and pregnancy should not be left too late. Would-be diabetic mothers should be advised to attend a special pre-conception consultation in order that extra efforts to maintain strict glycaemic control may be made. Strict glycaemic control will reduce the congenital malformation rate (Ylinen *et al.*, 1984).

(b) Diabetic management during pregnancy

Every effort should be made to maintain good glycaemic control. To this end the patient should be seen by the diabetologist every 2 weeks. There must be open access for advice via the telephone, the ward, the outpatients or day hospital. Education should continue with plenty of reassurance. The patient must be reassured particularly about her baby and that it will not be diabetic. The lower insulin requirement during the first 3 months of the pregnancy should be explained and the gradually increasing requirement particularly during the last 3 months should be anticipated. Patients should be taught how to adjust their own insulin and encouraged to do so. They should continue with a diet for healthy living (see dietary section).

It should be explained that the aim of managing diabetes during pregnancy is a full-term (40 weeks) normal vaginal delivery.

Home blood glucose monitoring using a meter should be introduced if this is not already used. The preprandial and fasting blood glucose levels should be maintained at between 3 and 7 mmol/1 (54 and 126 mg%) and 3–4 measurements made per day. The interval blood sugar measured by the laboratory should be checked every 2 months or as indicated. The haemoglobin A1 should be measured every 2 months and should be within the normal range set by the laboratory and the method used.

Such efforts to maintain normoglycaemia should increased the ease with which the patient becomes pregnant and in addition to this reduce the malformation rate.

(c) Obstetric management of the diabetic pregnancy

In diabetic pregnancy free from obstetric complications the aim should be a full-term or near-full-term (40 weeks) vaginal delivery. (Drury *et al.*, 1983).

There is a danger that routine over monitoring and fetal surveillance may concentrate the clinician's mind on the machinery and not the patient. This may lead to an unnecessarily high Caesarian section rate (it has risen to 60–80% in some centres). A surfeit of technology may generate uncertainty and encourage intervention (*Lancet*, 1985).

On the whole, if the patient has good glycaemic control, no evidence of microvascular disease, and no obstetric complications, she should be treated from the obstetric point of view in no way different from the non-diabetic.

(d) Delivery

Unnecessary Caesarian sections may do more harm than good. In a large group of patients with a Caesarian section rate of 20% the fetal mortality rate was 11%. In patients allowed to deliver normally at less than 38 weeks the mortality rate was 9.8%. However, if patients were delivered by the normal route with a gestation of equal to or greater than 38 weeks the mortality rate dropped to 2.4% (Drury, 1961).

In a well-controlled uncomplicated diabetic pregnancy there is also no need for the patient to be admitted for a period of observation prior to delivery. If the patient is admitted it must be for obstetric reasons or for reasons of poor diabetic control.

The delivery regimen should aim to avoid ketosis, hyperglycaemia and hypoglycaemia. The patient should maintain a high-fibre, high-carbohydrate intake prior to delivery and should take the insulin required to control blood glucose levels.

For a spontaneous delivery an i.v. infusion of 5% dextrose, 1 litre in 4–6 hours should be set up. Blood glucose levels should be monitored and controlled with a low dose intravenous insulin infusion (Human Actrapid or Neutral Soluble via a pump) at a rate of approximately 0.5 units per hour. This rate should be varied to control blood sugar levels at various stages of labour.

If induction is required then the treatment of the diabetes should be similar to that described.

For caesarian section a PIG regimen or a low-dose infusion of intravenous insulin should be used (see section 5.3).

Following delivery the patient's insulin requirement falls dramatically and must be anticipated to prevent hypoglycaemia. Infants of diabetic mothers should be cared for in a special Baby Unit until the initial dangers of the perinatal period are past (e.g. respiratory distress syndrome, hypoglycaemia, hypocalcaemia and hyperbilirubinaemia). The mother and child should be seen prior to discharge from hospital and again shortly after discharge (one month) to check glycaemic control and sort out any problems. However, frequent clinic attendance should not be expected as the new mother will be quite busy enough caring for her family. Continued home blood glucose monitoring should be encouraged and the patient advised to contact the clinic should any problems arise. Here a good relationship of trust between diabetologist and patient should exist and is invaluable. A firm follow-up appointment should be given for 4–6 months and, should the patient not attend further contact with the patient should be pursued with further appointments, a letter to the family doctor and if necessary a visit from the Diabetic Liaison Sister.

The successful outcome of a diabetic pregnancy depends upon hard work by doctors, nurses and above all by the patient.

REFERENCES AND FURTHER READING

Deckert, T., Poulsen, J.E. and Larsen, M. (1978) Prognosis of diabetes with diabetes onset before the age of 31. ii. Factors influencing the prognosis. *Diabetologia*, **14**, 371–77.

Drury, M.I., Strange, J.M., Foley, M.E. and MacDonald, D.W. (1983) Pregnancy in the diabetic patient : timing and mode of delivery. *Obstet. Gynaecol.*, **62**, 279–83.

Drury, M.I. (1961) Diabetes mellitus complicating pregnancy. *Irish J. Med. Sci*, **10**, 425–53.

Editorial (1985) *Lancet*, **i**, 961–62.

Fleming, P.C. (1985). What is happening to our diabetic patients? An audit of care in general practice. *Practical Diabetes*, **2**, 26–29.

Hammersley, M.S., Holland, M.R., Walford, S. and Thorne, P.A. (1985) What happens to defaulters from a diabetic clinic? *Br. Med. J.*, **291**, 1330–32.

Hayes, T.M. and Harries, J. (1984) Randomised control trial of routine hospital clinic care versus routine general practice care for type 2 diabetic. *Br. Med. J.*, **289**, 728–30.

Hill, R.D. (1976) Community care service for diabetics in the Poole area. *Br. Med. J.*, 1137–39.

Hill, R.D. (1984) *Computer Update*, **January 9th**.

Hill, R.D. (1986) Report of the B.D.A. Working Party on Computing in Diabetes. Published in *Practical Diabetes* as a series (1986).

Hoechst Meducation Service *Co-operation Record Book for Diabetic Patients*. Hoechst UK Pharmaceutical Division, Hoechst House, Salisbury Road, Hounslow, Middlesex TW4 6JH.

McCormack, M. (1976) Patient recall system. *Update*, **12**, 552.

Pedersen, J. (1977) In *The Pregnant Diabetic and Her Newborn*, 2nd edn. Munksgaard, Copenhagen.

Royal College of Physicians of London (Committee on Endocrinology and Diabetes) and British Diabetic Association (1984) *Report on the Provision of Medical Care for Adult Diabetic Patients in the United Kingdom*.

Russell, R.G., Canney, J.C., Simm, I.S.G., *et al.* (1974) *Update*, **8**, 945–54 (Diabetic Clinics in General Practice.)

Singh, B.M., Holland, M.R. and Thorne, P.A. (1984) Metabolic control of diabetes in general practice clinics: comparison with a hospital clinic. *Br. Med. J.*, **289**, 726–28.

Tasker, P.R.W. (1984) Is diabetes a disease for general practice? *Pract. Diabetes*, **1**, 21–24.

Thorne, P.A. and Russell, R.G. (1973) Diabetic clinics today and tomorrow: mini-clinics in general practice. *Br. Med. J.*, **ii**, 534.

Upton, C.E. (1975) Diabetic community care. *Practitioner*, **July**, 215.

White, P. (1965) Pregnancy and diabetes, medical aspects. *Med. Clin. N. Am.*, **49**, 1015–24.

Wilkes, E. and Laughton, E.E. (1980) The diabetic, the hospital, and primary care. *J. R. Coll. Gen. Pract.*, **30**, 199–206.

Ylinen, K., Aul, A.P., Stenman, U.H. Kesaniema, Kicokkanen, R. and Teroma, K. (1984) Risk of minor and major foetal malformation in diabetics with High HbA1 values in early pregnancy. *Br. Med. J.*, **289**, 345–6.

Yudkin, J.S., Boucher B.J., Schopflin, K.E. *et al.* (1980) The quality of diabetic care in a London health care district. *J. Epidemiol. Commun. Hlth.*, **34**, 277–80.

· Seven ·

Diabetic eye disease

R.D. Hill in association with Martin Crick FRCS (Ophthalmologist) and Ralph Goldenberg FBCO (Ophthalmic Optician)

7.1 INTRODUCTION

The detail contained in this chapter is a reflection of the importance of diabetic eye disease. Section 7.2 attempts to demonstrate the size of the problem. Sections 7.3 and 7.4 describe the essential structure and function of the eye and provide a basis for the understanding of the pathological processes and appearances. Section 7.5 stresses the importance of eye examination.

Section 7.6 describes the many and varied ocular manifestations of diabetes mellitus, putting diabetic retinopathy (7.7, 7.8, and 7.9) in perspective. Section 7.10 describes associated conditions.

Section 7.11 describes methods of documentation which are an essential part of the follow-up of a chronic and progressive condition.

Section 7.12 outlines the present methods of prevention and treatment available. Section 7.13 describes the organisation of health care necessary for the follow up of diabetic eye disease and 7.14 discusses the costs involved. In 7.15 a suggested plan of action is outlined for those wishing to set up an integrated service for the care of diabetic eye disease.

7.2 EPIDEMIOLOGY – THE SIZE OF THE PROBLEM

Table 7.1 shows the prevalence of diabetes, the overall prevalence of diabetic retinopathy, and the overall prevalence of serious retinopathy within the diabetic population. Serious retinopathy may be defined as retinopathy which is sight threatening and requiring immediate treatment. The prevalence figures are related to two units of population. A unit of 250 000 represents a population cared for by a large district general hospital in the United Kingdom and a unit of

Table 7.1 Prevalence of diabetic eye disease

Population unit	*Diabetes*	*Retinopathy*	*Serious retinopathy*	*Blind*
Prevalence	1.01%	26–35%	9.5–11%	1–2%
250 000	2525	657–884	240–278	25–51
2500	25	7–9	2–3	0–1

2500 represents a population cared for by a family doctor in the United Kingdom. The figure shows that for the 250 000 population unit, 2525 will have diabetes. Of these 657–844 will have retinopathy and 240–278 will have a potentially blinding retinopathy. For the population unit of 2500, 25 patients will have diabetes, 7–9 will have retinopathy and 2–3 will have potentially blinding disease.

Table 7.2 shows the expected incidence of diabetic eye disease. This gives some idea of the new cases of diabetic eye disease which might be seen per year in the two population units considered. Of the patients with diabetes 5% per annum might be expected to develop retinopathy. In the 250 000 population unit, 126 new cases of retinopathy might be discovered per annum. In the 2500 population unit only 1 new case of diabetic retinopathy will appear per annum. In the 250 000 population unit, 30 new cases of serious retinopathy per annum might be expected. In the 2500 population unit one patient every 3 years with serious retinopathy might be expected. This highlights the problem of screening for diabetic eye disease at the primary health care level. Because of the dilution of clinical material the family doctor will only have 25 diabetics to follow up. Within his diabetic population he might expect to have between 7–9 patients with retinopathy and 2 or 3 of these will have serious retinopathy. Only 1 new case of retinopthy will appear in his

Table 7.2 Incidence of diabetic eye disease

Population unit	*Diabetics at risk*	*Retinopathy*	*Serious retinopathy*
Incidence		5% PA	1.2% PA
250 000	2525	126 PA	30 PA
2500	25	1	1 every 3 years

practice per annum and only 1 patient every 3 years will present with serious retinopathy. Under these circumstances it would be only too easy for the family doctor to miss a retinopathy because of lack of clinical experience.

Table 7.3 shows the prevalence of diabetic retinopathy after 10 years duration of diabetes, in relation to the age of onset of diabetes. 7% of those whose diabetes started before the age of 20 will have retinopathy, compared with 10% of those who developed diabetes between 20 and 40 years. For those whose diabetes was diagnosed after the age of 40 the prevalence rises to 25%. Although these figures are interesting in that they show an increase in prevalence of retinopathy related to the age of onset of diabetes they are of no help in deciding who should or who should not should be examined for retinopathy. They do, however, indicate that with an ageing population the problem of retinopathy will increase.

Although the above figures may appear small in relation to the whole population and to the medical work load in general, it is important to realize that diabetes mellitus is the single most common cause of blindness in the 30–64-year-old age group in the United Kingdom.

The incidence of blind registration due to diabetes in the United Kingdom is 15 per million per year. Survey figures suggest that this is an underestimate. Patients appear to be reticent about registering as blind. The committee on Blindness Due to Diabetes of The British Diabetic Association considers that a figure of 30 per million population per year would be a more realistic figure.

If we are to reduce the incidence of blindness due to diabetic retinopathy then it is important to understand the condition in order that preventative measures may be taken, early detection achieved, and suitable treatment instituted.

Table 7.3 Prevalence of diabetic retinopathy after 10 years duration of diabetes in relation to age of onset

Age of onset	*Prevalence of retinopathy (%)*
Under 20	7
20–40	10
Over 40	25

The first step in understanding the ocular manifestations of diabetes is to understand the normal structure and function of the eye.

7.3 THE STRUCTURE OF THE EYE WITH PARTICULAR REFERENCE TO THE RETINA

Figure 7.1 shows diagramatically a horizontal section through the right eye. The light beam traverses the cornea, the anterior chamber (aqueous) and then passes through the pupil to the lens. From the lens it passes through the vitreous along the optical axis of the eye to be focused on the fovea. The fovea and the immediate area surrounding it (the macula) form the most sensitive part of the retina. In order to appreciate the nature of diabetic retinopathy it is important to understand the structure of the retina and the adjacent choroid.

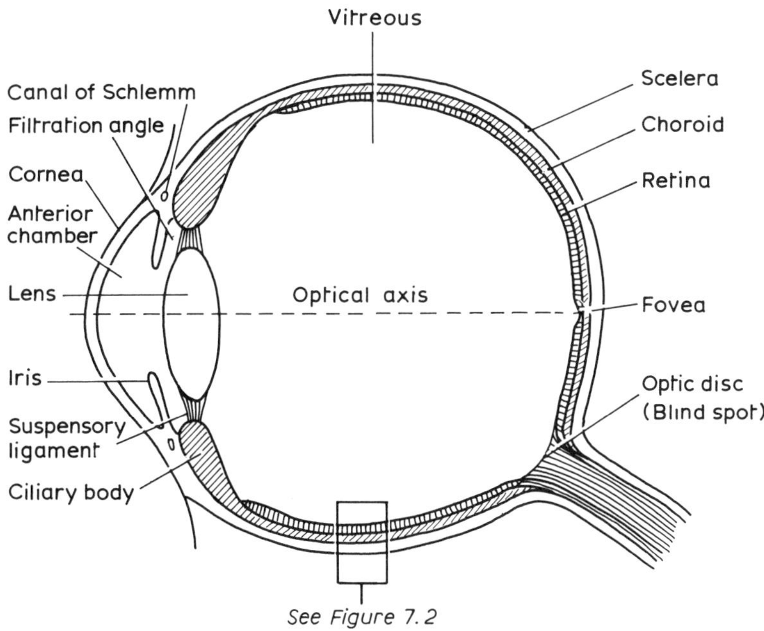

Figure 7.1 Structure of the eye. (Sclera, choroid and retina – thicknesses not drawn to scale.)

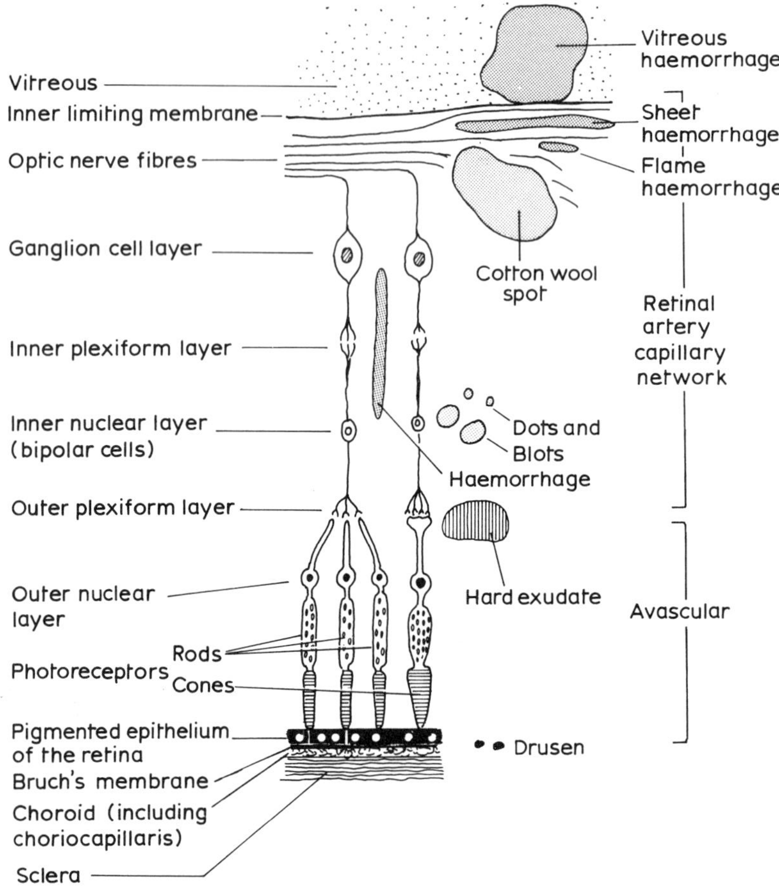

Figure 7.2 The structure of the retina and its pathology. Not drawn to scale.

Figure 7.2 diagrammatically represents the structure of the retina and the adjacent choroid. The shape of the eye and its whole structure is supported by the tough outer sclera. Between the sclera and the retina lies the choroid. The vascular supply to the choroid originates as branches from extracranial branches of the internal carotid artery. These vessels form a fine network of capillaries

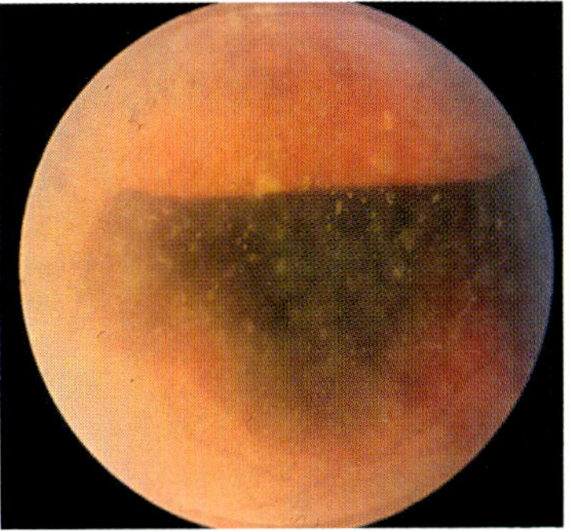
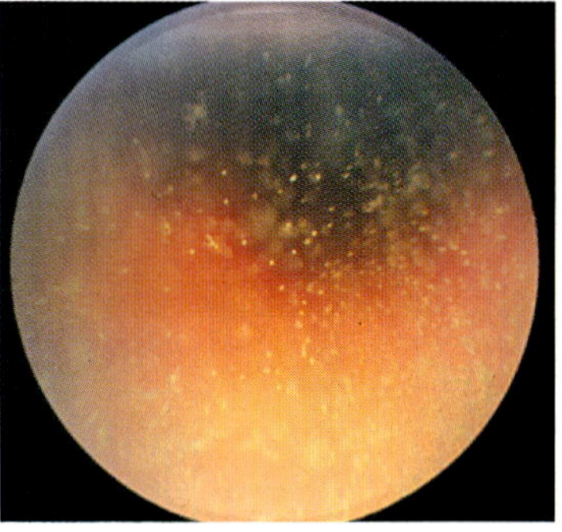

Plate 7 Sub-hyaloid haemorrhage and asteroid hyalosis. Patient aged 55 years, non-insulin dependent diabetes, proliferative retinopathy with haemorrhage. The fluid level of the sub-hyaloid haemorrhage may be seen at the top of the photograph (left). On the right the camera is focussed on the silver-white dots floating in the vitreous, i.e. asteroid hyalosis.

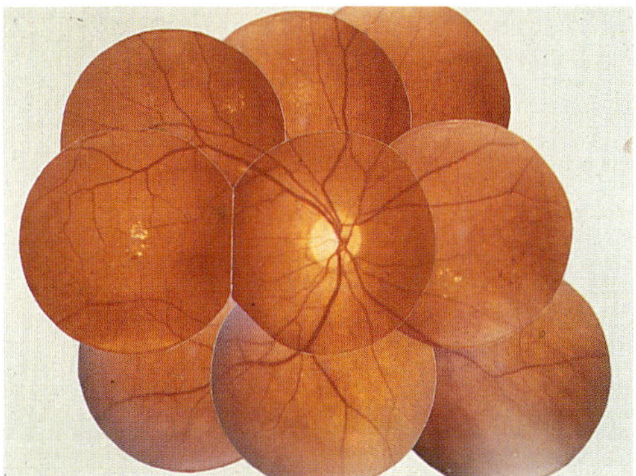

Plate 8 Montage of fundal photographs to demonstrate the importance of looking in the periphery of the retina for diabetic changes.

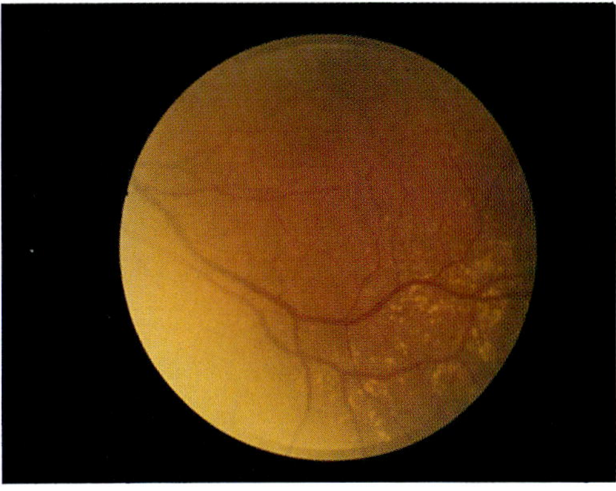

Plate 9 Drusen.

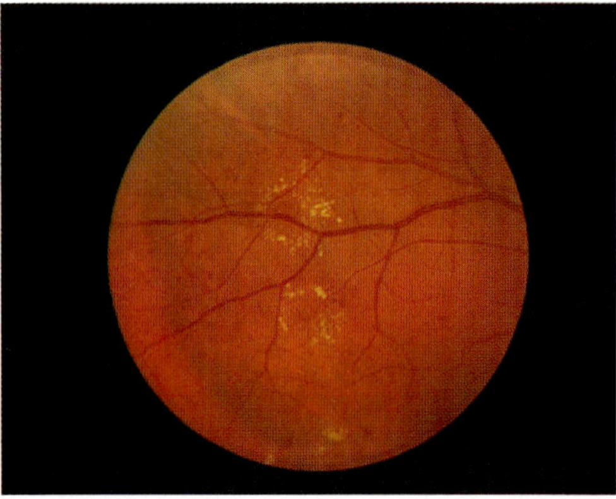

Plate 10 Background retinopathy. Dots, blots, hard exudates, circinate hard exudates and haemorrhages.

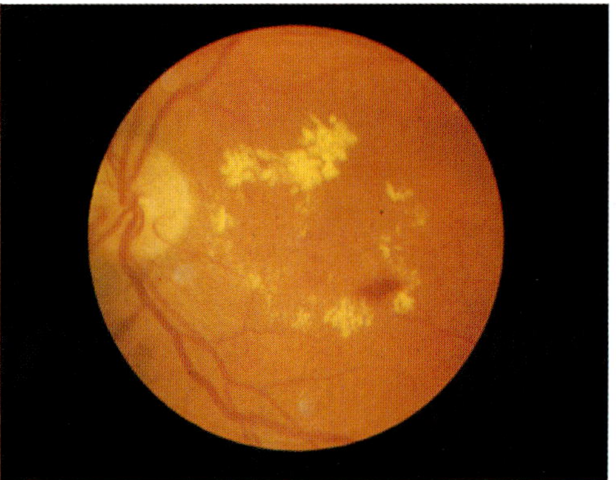

Plate 11 Exudative maculopathy. Patient aged 60 years. Presenting symptom poor visual acuity. Diagnosis made by ophthalmic optician.

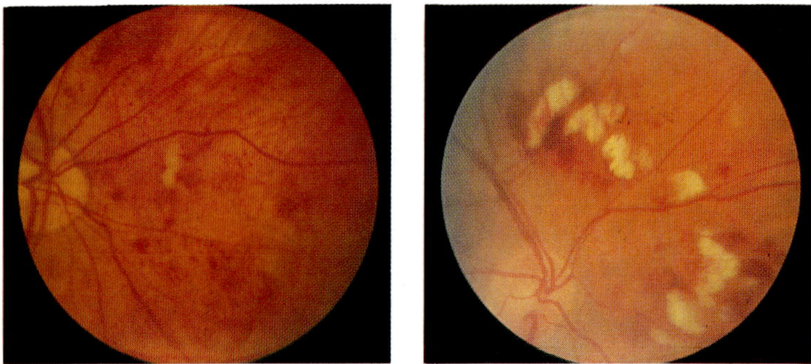

Plate 12 Background retinopathy with ischaemic features. Patient aged 45 years, insulin-dependent diabetes for 20 years. Condition discovered at routine screening for diabetic retinopathy. Photograph shows haemorrhagic retina with extensive cotton wool spots. This condition is pre-proliferative.

beneath the retina known as the choriocapillaris. This network of capillaries is separated from the photoreceptors by the pigment epithelium. The photoreceptors are of two types: the cones, which are sensitive to high-intensity light and give colour appreciation, and rods which are sensitive to low-intensity light but not to colours. The nuclei of the photoreceptor cells together form the outer nuclear layer. The cell processes of the photoreceptors then pass into the outer plexiform layer where synapses are formed with various cells in the retina and in particular with the dendrites of bipolar cells whose nuclei form the inner nuclear layer. The axonal processes of these cells synapse with the dendrites of the ganglion cells to form the inner plexiform layer. The ganglion cells are the cell bodies of the optic nerve. The axonal processes of the ganglion cells pass to the surface of the retina and then turn towards the optic disc lying beneath the inner limiting membrane which separates them from the hyaloid membrane of the vitreous body. The neurones sweep towards the optic disc where they form the optic nerve.

It is necessary to understand the vascular supply to the complex structure of the retina to be able to understand the nature of the retinopathic appearances in diabetes. The outer area of the retina from the chorioretinal pigment layer to the outer nuclear layer is avascular. It derives its nutrition by diffusion from the choriocapillaris lying outside the chorioretinal pigment layer.

The inner layer of the retina from the outer plexiform layer to the inner limiting membrane covering the neurovascular nerve layer is supplied with oxygen and nutrients by a capillary network derived from the retinal vessels. The retinal artery is a branch of the internal carotid artery. It passes into the optic nerve and emerges via the optic cup. The artery divides into four main vessels supplying the four quadrants of the eye. These are the superior nasal, inferior nasal, superior temporal and inferior temporal arteries (*Figure 7.3*). Blood in the capillary network derived from the retinal arteries and supplying the vascular part of the retina, is collected in a series of veins which come together to form the retinal veins. These lie in close relation, and are similar to the retinal arteries. The retinal veins pass to the optic disc and exit from the eye via the optic (physiological) cup.

In the area surrounding the fovea the vascular layer on the retina thins until at the fovea there only remains the avascular part of the

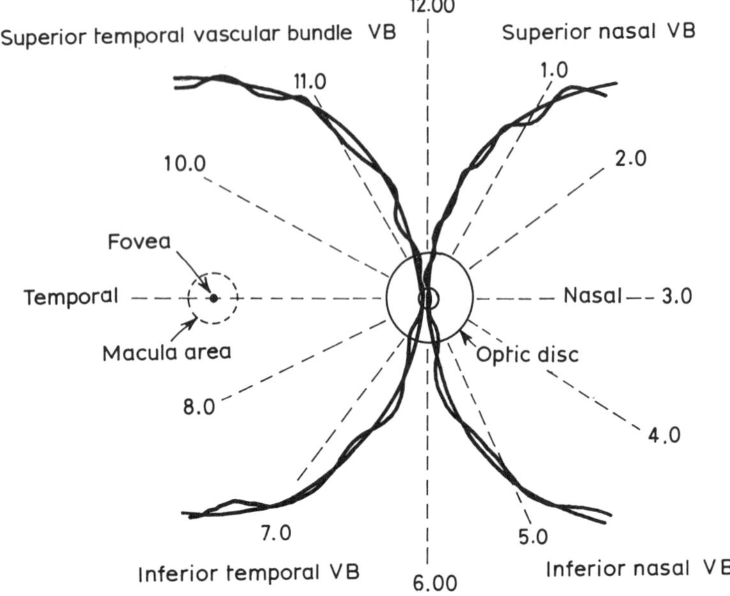

Figure 7.3 Structure of the retinal artery (right eye).

retina. This forms a dip which is seen as the macular reflex. The fovea thus receives the whole of its nutrition by diffusion from the choriocapillaris beneath the chorioretinal pigmented layer.

There is a very important difference between the capillaries arising from the retinal arteries and those of the choriocapillaris. The capillaries in the vascular part of the retina have endothelial cells with 'tight junctions'. These capillaries are similar to those capillaries supplying the brain. On the other hand, the endothelial cells of the choriocapillaris do not have 'tight junctions' and are similar to capillaries found anywhere else in the body. The tight junctions of the vascular layer prevent free diffusion. Any transport of substances from inside the capillary to the retina must therefore be by active transport. There is thus a blood-retinal barrier similar to the blood-brain barrier. On the other hand the vessels of the choriocapillaries, having no tight junctions, allow free diffusion from blood to the extracellular spaces. There are tight junctions between the cells of the pigment epithelium which control diffusion from the choriocapillaris into the avascular layer of the retina.

7.4 NORMAL FUNCTION OF THE EYE

Light rays entering the eye are refracted by the cornea and again by the lens to focus the image on the retina. The image is normally focused on the most sensitive part of the retina, the fovea. At the fovea the inner layers of the retina are thinned out and the area contains no capillaries. The image formed by the refracting system of the eye is therefore focused almost directly onto the photoreceptors of the fovea. One important consequence of this arangement is that the fovea receives its nutrition almost entirely by diffusion from the choriocapillaris and not from the vascular layer of the retina. The tightly packed photoreceptor cones allow the appreciation of both detail and colour. This is in contrast to the more peripheral parts of the retina which contain rods. These areas give less detailed information on images, do not give colour appreciation but are able to pick up light of low intensity.

Electrical impulses produced in the rods and cones are transmitted through synapses in the outer plexiform layer to the inner neurone nuclear layer. The impulses are then transmitted on through the inner plexiform layer synapses to the ganglion cells of the optic nerve. It will be noted that images focused on areas of the retina other than the fovea have to pass through the vascular layer of the retina before reaching the avascular layer of the retina containing the photoreceptors.

7.5 EXAMINATION OF THE EYE

The steps of eye examination are as follows:

1. Tell the patient what is to be done.
2. Measure distant visual acuity (DVA) (correction with either the patients DISTANT spectacles or a pinhole), Snellen type well lit. Distance 6 m or nearer, one eye at a time.
3. Measure reading vision – J. Type.
4. Measure intraocular pressure (IOP).
5. Dilate the pupil : (tropicamide, ½ – 1%.)
6. Direct ophthalmoscopy.
7. Other methods:
   (i) Indirect ophthalmoscopy.
   (ii) Slit lamp.

(iii) Retinal photography.
(iv) Fluoroscein angiography.

The patient must be told what is to be done and why the examination is being carried out. This is an opportunity to continue patient education which must not be missed.

The distant visual acuity (DVA) should be measured using a well-lit Snellen chart at a distance of 6 m. The acuity should be measured one eye at a time and corrected with the patient's distant spectacles if worn. Ophthalmologists and ophthalmic opticians are able to correct refractive errors but in the general medical clinic or family doctor's consulting room a 'pinhole' may be used. If the patient is asked to look through a small pinhole in a card at the Snellen type the visual acuity will be corrected by several lines on the chart. This is because only the centre part of the refracting system along the optical axis is used. The use of the 'pinhole' improves distant vision but may make the visual acuity worse in the presence of central lens opacity. It is therefore useful in distinguishing this type of disorder from simple refractive errors. If the patient is not able to read the largest symbol on Snellen type at 6 m the distance should be shortened at metre intervals until such time as the type can be read. If the largest type cannot be seen at a distance of 2 m then a further assessment of visual acuity may be made by asking the patient to count fingers at a distance of 1 m. If not able to do this the patient may be able to detect hand movements at 1 m. If the patient cannot appreciate hand movements then a light should be shone into the eye to determine whether the patient has light perception.

Central vision (mascular function) may also be assessed by measuring the near visual acuity. The vision should be tested one eye at a time using the patient's reading spectacles if necessary. Amsler or J-type should be used in a good light and held at a comfortable distance (around 40 cm).

When measuring either distance or near visual acuity it is an advantage to be able to correct refractive errors. Here the ophthalmologist, ophthalmalic medical practitioner and ophthalmic optician have an advantage over the physician.

Different Snellen type charts are available for the illiterate or patients with a language problem and also for children.

If possible the intraocular pressure should be measured. This measurement is usually only undertaken by ophthalmologists, ophthalmic medical practitioners and ophthalmic opticians.

The pupil should be dilated with tropicamide ½–1%. Patients with brown eyes usually require the higher concentration. Patients should be warned that the effect of the drops will last approximately 3 hours. It is not necessary to reverse the effect with Pilocarpine. Although the mydriatic will produce some blurring of near vision it should not significantly affect distant vision. However, the patients should be warned to take care when driving. Mydriatics should not be used in patients with known glaucoma or previous eye surgery. It is better to refer these patients to an ophthalmologist for screening.

The danger of precipitating closed angle glaucoma by the use of mydriatics is negligible.

A good ophthalmoscope is essential for the successful examination of the eye. Its lens system should be clean and its light source bright. The frequent replacement of batteries is essential. 'Seeing through a glass darkly' has no place in ophthalmoscopic examination! There are many good instruments on the market. It is recommended that the lens system should provide a minimum adjustment of plus 10 – minus 10 diopters. It is an advantage to have a system of additional lens interposition for patients with a large refraction defect (i.e. high myopes or patients with a large hypermetrophic defect). A halogen light source together with rechargeable batteries have a considerable advantage over the old conventional light system. It is also an advantage to have a variable light beam size. By adjusting the beam of light to enter the pupil to gain maximum illumination with minimal reflection from the cornea and iris a clearer picture of the retina will be obtained. This is particularly important when examining the macular area and a macular spot is invaluable. In the author's view the Keeler Specialist ophthalmoscope is second to none. However, what is important is that the operator must get to know his own instrument and by constant practice use it efficiently.

It is preferable to examine the eye in a darkened room.

A small light source on which the patient can fix his gaze during the eye examination makes life easier for the observer.

Examination of the eye should begin with the ophthalmoscope lens system set to + 10 diopters. Light should be shone into the eye from a distance of approximately 10 cm and the red reflex through the pupil observed. Any lens opacities will stand out as black areas (Plates 4 and 5). The lens systems should then be adjusted in a minus direction and close inspection of the cornea, the surrounding sclera, the anterior chamber, the iris, and the lens made. By adjusting the lens system in a stepwise fashion the vision may be focused at greater and greater depths into the eye passing through the lens into the vitreous and thence down to the disc. If important physical signs are not to be missed it is essential to be obsessional about carrying out the eye examination. Unless these steps are taken such important signs as new vessels in the iris (Plate 6), lens opacities, and interesting though not dangerous conditions such as asteroid hyalosis (hyalatis, plate 7) will be missed.

On reaching the disc this should be brought sharply into focus. The characteristics of the disc, its outline, its colour and the optic cup should be observed. It is often possible to see the cribriform plate at the bottom of the optic disc. The disc should be carefully examined for the presence of abnormal vessels and then each of the four main vascular bundles should be examined in turn (superior nasal, inferior nasal, superior temple, inferior temple).

The retina should then be examined systematically moving out from the disc to the periphery in a stepwise fashion as if examining the face of a clock from the spindle to the numbers (*Figure 7.3*). Thus the eye should travel from the disc to 1 o'clock back to the disc, then out to 2 o'clock back to the disc, then out to 3 o'clock back to the disc, and so on. By doing this the whole of the retina will be observed and no part missed. To examine the extremes of the peripheral part of the retina in the temporal area it is often necessary to ask the patient to look laterally. Good dilatation is essential if the peripheral part of the retina is to be examined adequately. The observer may be surprised to find that an apparently normal fundus has extensive retinopathy in the periphery (Plate 8).

Finally the beam size should be reduced to the minimum (macula spot) and the patient asked to look at the ophthalmoscope light. This will enable the observer to examine the macula area in detail. This part of the examination should be left until last as the brightness of the light impinging upon the macula area often induces photophobia.

Direct ophthalmoscopy provides an upright image of the retina with a magnification of times 16. However, as only a uniocular view is obtained of the retina depth is difficult to appreciate. Indirect ophthalmoscopy gives an inverted image with a magnification of times 4. This allows a wide view of the retina and the binocular view gives an appreciation of depth. Indirect ophthalmoscopy is usually only carried out by ophthalmologists.

If necessary further examination of the eye can be carried out using a slit lamp, retinal photography, or fluoroscein angiography.

There are certain variations in retinal appearance which may confuse the inexperienced:

1. Variation in pigmentation – Asian, Caucasian, Negroid.
2. Choroid vessels.
3. Choroiditis – laser burns and toxoplamosis.
4. Drusen. (Plate 9.)
5. Senile macula degeneration.
6. Opaque nerve fibres.

A great deal of this variation depends on the amount of pigment in the pigmented epithelium of the retina. If pigmentation is deficient then the choroidal vessels may be seen through the retina and confusion caused. Choroidal vessels may be distinguished by their random distribution which does not follow the normal pattern of the retinal vasculature. The loss of pigment may be generalized as in racial differences, or localized. The latter abnormality may be congenital or familial but is also seen following localized choroiditis due to toxoplasma or laser burns (Plate 8). Localized areas of choroiditis are often surrounded by clumped pigment.

Increased amount of pigment may also be of racial origin (Negroid races).

Areas of degeneration in Bruch's membrane (*Figure 7.2*) produce localized small rounded yellow-white lesions called Drusen (Plate 9). These may be solitary or diffuse and are not related to diabetes. They may be confused with hard exudates.

An apparently normal retina associated with poor central vision may be due to senile macular degeration. An ophthalmological opinion should be sought for confirmation.

7.6 THE OCULAR MANIFESTATIONS OF DIABETES MELLITUS

The ocular manifestations of diabetes may be summarized as follows:

Early:
1. Transient refractory changes.
2. Diabetic cataract. (Plate 4.)

Late:
1. Accelerated senile cataract. (Plate 5.)
2. Diabetic retinopathy and its complications.
3. Oculomotor palsies.

Complications of diabetic retinopathy:
1. Maculopathy.
2. Vitreous haemorrhage/membrane formation.
3. Traction retinal detachment.
4. Rubeotic glaucoma. (Plate 6.)

The osmolarity of the blood and tissue fluids changes with the rise and fall of blood glucose concentrations. Changes in osmolarity produce changes in the refractory media of the eye. Transient errors of refraction are therefore produced. Hyperglycaemia produces myopia. This is corrected as the blood glucose falls to normal. If a patient is treated with insulin and there is a rapid fall in blood glucose concentration then hypermetropia may develop. This is usually transient. The practical importance of the transient refractory changes associated with hyper- and hypoglycaemia must not be underestimated. Patients must be warned not to have their eyes refracted and spectacles prescribed until the blood glucose is stable. To have spectacles prescribed before the correction of hyperglycaemia can be an expensive error.

Rarely young patients with insulin-dependent diabetes develop lens opacities which are clearly visible on examination. The normal pathway for glucose metabolism in the lens is that of glucose oxidiation starting with the enzyme hexokinase and eventually finishing with the production of carbon dioxide and water. This pathway is fully saturated at normal blood glucose concentrations. However, an alternative pathway for glucose metabolism does exist. This is known as the sorbitol pathway. The enzyme aldose reductase initiates the series of events which culminates in the production of the alcohol sorbitol. Sorbitol is slowly metabolized and cannot diffuse out of the cell. This pathway is unsaturated at normal blood glucose concentrations. With the increasing blood glucose concentrations of diabetes mellitus the hexokinase–glycolytic pathway cannot increase its activity. However, the sorbitol pathway increases its activity and sorbitol collects in the cell. Because of the slow metabolism of the sorbitol and because sorbitol cannot diffuse out of the cell, the high concentrations of sorbitol reached damage the internal structure of the cell. The intracellular osmolarity increases and the cells begin to swell. The loss of the ordered regular structure of the lens produces severe refractory errors and the patient complains of a marked decrease in visual acuity. Examination at this time may show the typical 'snowflake' appearance of diabetic cataract (Plate 4). With good diabetic control some of these cataracts disappear and visual acuity is restored. However, the damage to the lens may be permanent and necessitate cataract extraction.

In contrast to the rarity of the diabetic cataract accelerated senile cataract is very common. The mechanism of lens damage is unknown. However, it may be similar to the one described above but over a long period of time. Cataracts of this type are usually initially situated in the peripheral parts of the lens and have the appearance of roman numerals on a clock face (Plate 5). Initially visual acuity is spared since the optical axis of the lens is not affected. However, as time passes the blocks of lens opacity expand and eventually diminish the visual acuity. Other types of cataract may appear in the absence of typical roman numeral cataract. These may be situated on the optical axis of the eye, particularly at the posterior pole. When this occurs even a small opacity produces a marked diminution in visual acuity.

Because of the possible part the sorbitol plays in the development of cataract it has been suggested that aldose reductase inhibitors may have a part to play in the treatment of prevention of cataract in diabetes. However, this is for the future and at present the only treatment available is surgical. Surgical treatment of cataracts should not be undertaken and the patient should not be referred to an ophthalmologist until such time as the visual acuity in both eyes warrants the treatment of one eye. However, in very well controlled diabetics a lens implant may be considered and earlier referral is therefore justified.

Diabetic retinopathy and its complications are dealt with in detail below.

Diabetic mononeuritis affecting the nerves supplying the external ocular muscles is not an uncommon condition afflicting the elderly. It is sometime accompanied by pain in the face or forehead and may be very distressing, producing severe diplopia. However, it is fortunate that these ocular palsies are transient and recover in a matter of weeks or months. The patient may be encouraged that full recovery should take place.

7.7 DIABETIC RETINOPATHY – PATHOGENESIS

The features of diabetic retinopathy are a consequence of microvascular disease affecting the retina. The capillaries of the vascular part of the retina consist of basement membrane tubes lined with endothelial cells. As indicated earlier endothelial cells have tight junctions and prevent free diffusion from the lumen of the capillary via the basement membrane to the extracellular spaces of the retina. Any movement in this direction must be by active transport. Within the basement membrane there are embedded cells intimately concerned with its function. These are the pericytes. Perhaps the earliest manifestation of microvascular disease is the loss of the pericyte with endothelial proliferation and later endothelial loss. Capillaries affected in this way may form aneurismal dilatations (microaneurysms), non-endothelialized basement membrane tubes, or undergo complete closure. Damaged capillaries lose their tight junctions and exude plasma into the extracellular spaces. This produces retinal oedema and eventually lipid-rich precipitates are deposited in the retina having the appearance known as hard exudates (*Figure* 7.2, Plates 10 and 11). Thrombosis of microaneurysms and closure of capillaries result in severe retinal ischaemia. Normal axoplasmic flow within the nerves is halted and axoplasm collects in the ischaemic area. This has a whitish grey appearance of the so-called 'cotton wool spot' (*Figure* 7.2, Plate 12). Although cotton wool spots do not delineate the exact area of infarction (since the area of retinal infarction may be much larger) they always indicate retinal infarction. Another name for such lesions is 'soft exudate' which is perhaps better discarded.

Initially capillaries and arterioles may be dilated, perhaps in response to areas of retinal ischaemia. These abnormal areas may be seen in the retina as 'intraretinal microvascular abnormalities' (IRMA). Metabolic substances produced by the ischaemic retina may have a damaging affect on both arterioles and veins. Both become dilated and leak when crossing ischaemic non perfused areas of retina.

The hypothetical chemical messenger (or messengers) coming from ischaemic retina may be the stimulus to the production of new vessels. New vessels may grow out from the disc or from the vascular layer of the retina and even from the choroid. Initially these vessels have no supporting connective tissue. They do not have tight junctions and may be seen to leak profusely on fluoroscein angiography. The development of new vessels is called neovascularization (Plates 13,14 and15). Initially these may be intraretinal, i.e. in the vascular layer of the retina, but may eventually extend out onto the surface of the retina producing extra-retinal neovascularization. Initially these new vessels may lie flat on the surface of the retina but are later pulled forwards by detachment of the vitreous and later still white fibrous tissue develops producing the typical appearance of retinitis proliferans (Plate 16). Further contraction of the vitreous may produce retinal detachment by traction on the new vessels.

Damaged capillaries, microaneurysms, and new vessels may bleed. Haemorrhage occurring deep in the vascular layer of the retina tends to be confined between neural cells as they stream towards the inner surface of the retina. They therefore have a round appearance. They may be small and indistinguishable from microaneurysms which may be either thrombosed or be patent. Because of the uncertain nature of these lesions on ophthalmoscopy they are called 'dots' (Plate 10). Haemorrhages occurring in the inner nuclear layer (which is vertically orientated), form a red cell column between the neuronal layers which is seen end on and therefore appears round. These are known as 'blot' haemorrhages' (*Figure 7.2*, and Plate 10).

Superficial, 'flame-shape' haemorrhages arise from the superficial plexus of capillaries in the nerve layer. The flame-shape is produced by tracking of blood along and between the neurones as they stream towards the optic disc.

Preretinal new vessels produce retrohyaloid haemorrhages with a fluid level (Plate 7).

New vessels may bleed into the vitreous producing a diffuse vitreous haemorrhage (Plates 7 and 17).

New vessels extending forward into the iris may invade the filtration angle eventually producing rubeotic glaucoma (Plate 6).

Figure 7.2 represents schematically the position of the lesions of diabetic retinopathy within the retina.

7.8 DIABETIC RETINOPATHY – DEFINITION OF RETINAL APPEARANCES

See Plates 6, 7 and 9–18. The retinal appearances defined in this section are as follows:

1. Dots.
2. Blots.
3. Hard exudates.
4. Capillary closure.
5. Cotton wool spots.
6. New vessels (proliferative retinopathy).
7. Venous changes.
8. Arterial changes.
9. Haemorrhages (other than 'blots'):
   (i) Flame shaped.
   (ii) Boat shaped.
   (iii) Diffuse
   (iv) Vitreous.
   (v) Deep dark round haemorrhages.
10. Maculopathy.

Although retinal appearances may be described in many ways the following definitions have proved very useful in practice.

When observing the individual components of the retinopathy, particular attention should be paid to the shape, the sharpness of outline, the colour, the size and other associated features.

1. Dots. These are small round red lesions. They have sharp clear outlines of a size less than the diameter of the superior temporal retinal artery as it crosses the disc margin. Dots may be produced by microaneurysms which are patent and thus have blood flow, by thrombosed microaneurysms, or by microhaemorrhages. These lesions are indistinguishable except by fluoroscein angiography. It is only possible to see lesions greater than 30 μm in diameter using ordinary ophthalmoscopy. However, fluoroscein angiography reveals lesions from 12 to 100 μm in diameter.
2. Blots. These are medium-sized round red lesions with less clear edges (like a blot of ink on blotting paper). The size is less than of the diameter of the optic disc (approximately 1500 μm). These are haemorrhages.

3. Hard exudates. These are irregular areas of white or yellowish white deposits with a clear sharp outline. They are often arranged in circinate patterns though they also occur in irregular patches. These arise from leaking vessels which produce retinal oedema. Retinal oedema may not be apparent on ordinary ophthalmoscopy but may be seen on slit lamp examination with a Rhuby lens. Hard exudates must be clearly distinguished from colloid bodies which are small round yellowish berry-like lesions not related to diabetes (Drusen).
4. Capillary closure. Capillary closure is suggested by a dull atropic appearance of the retina. An area of capillary closure may be suspected by the presence of surrounding dilated capillaries, microaneurysms, haemorrhages, and cotton wool spots. The areas may not be apparent to the inexperienced or even the experienced observer but can be shown on fluoroscein angiography.
5. Cotton wool spots. These appear as white or grey areas mainly distributed in the posterior pole of the retina. They have indistinct outlines but may be surrounded by haemorrhage, dilated capillaries or large microaneurysms. They are found in the neurovascular layer of the retina and become less common in the peripheral retina as the neuronal layer becomes thinner. Cotton wool spots are often associated with other signs of retinal ischaemia including intraretinal microvascular abnormalities, venous dilatation, venous beading and looping.
6. New vessels. The presence of either disc new vessels or peripheral new vessels indicate that the retinopathy has progressed to a proliferative stage which is sight threatening. The early detection of new vessels may be very difficult. They are usually a fine tangled mass of vessels of anomalous distribution. They may arise from the disc or in the periphery of the retina. New vessels are often associated with other signs of retinal ischaemia (capillary closure, IRMA, deep dark round haemorrhages, sheet haemorrhages, cotton wool spots, and venous abnormalities). If any doubt exists a fluoroscein angiogram will demonstrate massive leakage of fluoroscein from new vessels.
7. Venous changes. Slight venous dilatation occurs at diagnosis and at any time when metabolic control is poor. However, gross venous dilatation with irregularity, beading, and even looping indicate a severely ischaemic retina. Leakage of fluoroscein can

be demonstrated especially where such veins cross ischaemic non-perfused areas.

8. Arterial changes. Arteries show an irregularity of their diameter and wall sheathing. Often little is left of an artery apart from a white wall with a thin red column of blood. Arterioles crossing ischaemic areas may be dilated and on fluoroscein angiography may show massive leakage of fluoroscein.
9. Haemorrhages (other than blots). Haemorrhages are red lesions described on the basis of their shape and area covered:

   (i) Flame-shaped haemorrhages are as the name implies flame shaped. They lie in the neuronal layer between nerve fibres as they course towards the disc.

   (ii) Boat-shaped haemorrhages have a fluid level. They lie between the posterior surface of the vitreous and the retina.

   (iii) Diffuse haemorrhages are superficial, often irregular, and often extensive. They indicate severe ischaemic disease.

   (iv) Vitreous haemorrhages are diffuse haemorrhages within the vitreous which obscure a view of the retina. Vitreous haemorrhages indicate bleeding from new vessels.

   (v) Deep dark round haemorrhages are circular haemorrhages with a clear-cut sharp outline which are dark red and lie deep in the retina. These lesions may be associated with retinal ischaemia.
10. Maculopathy. This is defined as a decrease in visual acuity secondary to macular disease. It may be distinguished from an error of refraction in that the latter is improved with a pinhole whereas maculopathy is not improved. Diabetic maculopathy may be ischaemic or exudative. The presence of an exudative maculopathy may be inferred from the presence of hard exudates in the vicinity of the macula. Hard exudates, particularly if in a circinate arrangement, indicate extensive retinal oedema. Retinal oedema is difficult to see with an ordinary ophthalmoscope but may be demonstrated by the slit lamp. Fluoroscein angiography confirms leaking vessels affecting the macula.

    Definition of 'near' or 'within the vicinity of' the macula. This is defined as a lesion lying within an area of a circle approximately 7–800 μm in diameter centred on the fovea centralis. This is approximately a circle having a diameter equal to half that of the optic disc. Conveniently this is also the size of the macula spot of the Keeler specialist ophthalmoscope.

7.9 THE CLASSIFICATION OF DIABETIC RETINOPATHY AND ITS SIGNIFICANCE

The bringing together of the multiple manifestations of diabetic retinopathy into broad groups helps to focus the mind on their significance in relation to visual prognosis, the need for follow-up and indications for treatment. *Table 7.4* indicates the broad subdivisions into which diabetic retinopathy may be divided.

At least 26% of all patients with diabetes will show some manifestation of diabetic retinopathy on ophthalmoscopic examination. Of those patients showing retinopathy, 27.4% will have **simple background retinopathy**. On ophthalmoscopy these patients will

Table 7.4 The classification of diabetic retinopathy on ophthalmoscopy

		Prevalence in retinopathy population (%)
1. Simple background retinopathy (dots and blots only)		27.4
2. Exudative retinopathy (dots, blots and hard exudates only)		17.8
3. Preproliferative retinopathy (ischaemic retinopathy) dots, blots and cotton wool spots, with or without hard exudates or dots, blots, with or without hard exudates but with ischaemic features, e.g. capillary closure, deep dark round haemorrhages, sheet haemorrhages, IRMA, venous abnormalities		43.8
4. Proliferative retinopathy		11.0
Peripheral new vessels only (PNV)	40.6	
Disc new vessels only (DNV)	18.7	
PNV and DNV	6.8	
New vessels and fibrous proliferation	33.9	
5. Maculopathy (ischaemic or exudative)		16.4

show dots and blots only.

In addition to dots and blots 17.8% of patients will have hard exudates without any other features of retinopathy. This is **exudative retinopathy**.

The presence of cotton wool spots in 20.6% of the eyes with retinopathy indicate definite retinal ischaemia with infarction. However, the neural layer becomes thinner in the periphery and cotton wool spots may not appear despite severe ischaemia and retinal infarction. The presence of other ischaemic (features) such as widespread capillary closure (the retina has an atrophic, lack lustre, featureless appearance but this is best seen on fluorescein angiography), deep dark round haemorrhages, intraretinal microvascular abnormalities (IRMA) and venous abnormalities such as irregularity, tortuosity, beading and looping, all indicate retinal ischaemia. This is **preproliferative retinopathy**. Ischaemic retinopathy is seen in 43.8% of the retinopathic population.

Proliferative retinopathy is seen in 11% of those patients with a retinopathy. Of those patients with proliferative retinopathy 40.6% have peripheral new vessels only, 18.7% have disc new vessels only and 6.8% have both disc new vessels and peripheral new vessels. Nearly 40% have a combination of new vessels and fibrous proliferation. The development of retraction and eventual traction detachment leads to end stage diabetic eye disease.

Vitreous haemorrhage may complicate the picture of proliferative retinopathy at any time during its development.

Of all those patients with diabetic retinopathy 16.4% will have diminished visual acuity due to disease of the macula. This may be either due to ischaemia (ischaemic maculopathy) or retinal oedema (exudative maculopathy).

7.9.1 The evolution of diabetic retinopathy and its prognostic significance for visual acuity

Simple background retinopathy is the expected finding after 15–20 years of insulin dependent diabetes. However, 10% of patients with non insulin dependent diabetes will be found to have background retinopathy at the time of diagnosis. Indeed some patients may present with the diagnosis of exudative retinopathy as their first symptomatic feature of diabetes. Those diabetics who present with or are found to have retinopathy at the time of diagnosis are thought

Table 7.5 Diabetic retinopathy – risk of progression over 5 year period

Age of onset of diabetes (years)	*Microaneurysms (MA) only (%)*	*MA with hard exudates (%)*
<30	0	4
30–59	12	24

to have had diabetes for many years before the diagnosis was established. However, there are rare cases of severe and blinding retinopathy discovered at diagnosis in young insulin-dependent diabetics. It is difficult to believe that these patients had diabetes for any significant length of time before the diagnosis was established.

The risk of progression from good vision to blindness is dependent to some extent on the age of onset of the diabetes and the type of retinopathy (*Table 7.5*). For diabetes presenting under the age of 30 years with only microaneurysms present the chances of developing a significant sight threatening retinopathy in the next 5 years is practically nil. However, if an exudative retinopathy is present 4% of patients will progress to a sight-threatening retinopathy (maculopathy).

For those diabetics presenting between the ages of 30 and 59 years, 12% of those patients with microaneurysms only are likely to develop a sight-threatening retinopathy during the next 5 years. However, if there is an exudative retinopathy present then no less than 24% of patients will progress to severe loss of visual acuity.

The risk of developing severe visual impairment in the 2 years following the discovery of peripheral new vessels is between 6.8 and 29.7%. The risk is dependent on the presence of other risk factors such as the extent of the new vessels and the presence of vitreous or pre-retinal haemorrhages.

The risk of developing severe visual impairment in the 2 years following the discovery of disc new vessels is between 10.5 and 36.9%. Again this is dependent on the presence of other risk factors such as vitreous haemorrhage, pre-retinal haemorrhage and the extent of the new vessel growth.

The presence of multiple cotton wool spots is highly suggestive that the patient will develop new vessels within 2 years. This is why ischaemic retinopathy is classified as pre-proliferative.

Very rarely proliferative retinopathy undergoes spontaneous resolution. However, the 5-year blindness rate for patients with untreated proliferative retinopathy is about 60%.

The great danger of proliferative retinopathy is the development of a vitreous haemorrhage; 30% of patients with untreated proliferative retinopathy who have a vitreous haemorrhage are blind within 1 year.

Features which suggest that background retinopathy is progressing to proliferative retinopathy are as follows:

1. Capillary closure (non-perfusion).
2. Atrophic retina.
3. Multiple cotton wool spots.
4. Large sheet haemorrhages.
5. Deep dark round haemorrhages.
6. Venous looping and beading.
7. Arterial sheathing.
8. IRMA.

A rapidly progressive 'florid' retinopathy is fortunately only rarely seen. This has been described as 'rapid, bloody and blinding'. The patient is usually less that 35 years old, has widespread capillary dilatation with many microaneurysms. Large areas of capillary closure are seen with multiple cotton wool spots and haemorrhages. There is a rapid progression to new vessel formation, vitreous haemorrhage and blindness within 2 years.

Fortunately, diabetic retinopathy is only slowly progressive in most cases. The development of retinal oedema with hard exudates and maculopathy results in a gradual loss of visual acuity. However, the slowly progressive occlusive retinopathy with the eventual production of neovascularisation is asymptomatic until a vitreous haemorrhage produces sudden loss of vision.

7.9.2 Factors affecting the evolution of diabetic retinopathy

These are as follows:

1. Age.
2. Age of onset of diabetes.

3. Duration of diabetes.
4. Hypertension.
5. Chronic renal failure (diabetic nephropathy).
6. Glycaemic control (?).
7. Serum lipids (?).
8. Smoking (?).
9. Pregnancy/contraceptive pill (?).
10. Genetic factors (?).

Age, age of onset of diabetes, duration of diabetes, the presence of hypertension, and the presence of chronic renal failure, all affect the development of diabetic retinopathy adversely. Good glycaemic control may prevent or slow the evolution of retinopathy in the early stages. However, there is no evidence that tight diabetic control improves the prognosis for visual acuity once the disease has become established. There is even some evidence that very tight diabetic control can accelerate the rate of deterioration in vision.

The lowering of serum lipids is associated with a decrease in hard exudates in the retina. However, the disappearance of the lipid deposits does not alter the visual acuity.

Smoking may adversely affect ischaemic retinopathy but there are no definite figures on this.

During pregnancy a retinopathy may stay quiescent, get better, or get worse.

It is clear from what has been written that there must be many unknown factors operating in those patients developing or not developing retinopathy and that some of these may well be genetic.

7.10 ASSOCIATED CONDITIONS

Some of the conditions associated with diabetes are as follows:

1. Retinal vein/branch vein occlusion.
2. Asteroid hyalosis.
3. Glaucoma.
4. Lipaemia retinalis.
5. Xanthelasma.
6. Arcus senilis.

Retinal vein and retinal branch vein occlusion are more common in patients with diabetes and hypertension. The appearances may be very similar to diabetic retinopathy but a localized area of change particularly if uniocular should make one suspicious and look for the occluded vein.

Asteroid hyalosis (hyalitis) will be missed unless the eye is carefully examined by starting at the anterior chamber and working through focusing at a gradually increasing depth down towards the disc. As the name infers, this is a star-like appearance occurring in the vitreous. Silver, white or yellowish-white stars twinkle out of red sky when viewed with the ophthalmoscope. If the vitreous is fluid then the stars move about when the patient shakes the head. The appearances are rather like those of the child's snow scene toy which consists of a scene contained in a glass bubble containing fluid and a precipitate of white material. When the bubble is shaken the white flakes float down on the scene. The material deposited in the vitreous is almost certainly lipid (calcium soaps) in nature. This pretty appearance fortunately does not appear to have any clinical significance.

Chronic glaucoma is said to be more common in diabetics than in non-diabetics. The elevated intraocular pressure produces deep cupping of the optic disc with a gradual loss of peripheral vision. Sadly the patient may be asymptomatic until a severe loss of vision has occurred and the patient has 'tunnel' vision. This condition is both blinding and treatable. Between 1 and 2% of the population develop glaucoma. It is responsible for 13% of all blind registrations in the UK. By annual screening with the measurement of intraocular presssure as part of the examination, this condition should be removed from the list of causes of blindness in diabetes. Patients found to have signs of glaucoma or a raised intraocular pressure should be referred to an ophthalmologist without delay.

Lipaemia retinalis describes the creamy yellow milky appearance of the vessels and retina on ophthalmoscopy. This rare condition is due to the presence of turbid serum rich in triglycerides. This condition sometimes occurs with hyper-triglyceridaemia in poorly controlled diabetics. The appearances disappear with the return of blood lipids to normal.

The presence of xanthalasma and arcus suggests hypercholesterolaemia or other hyperlipidaemia. Both are said to be more common in patients with diabetes. Both are rather poor diagnostic signs. However, their presence should prompt an assessment of the blood lipids and appropriate treatment where necessary.

7.11 DOCUMENTATION

The main problem with diabetic clinic records is their size. Diabetes mellitus is a chronic disease and records accumulate over many years. The notes become bulky and disorganized and it is often impossible to trace any coherent theme running through them.

Eye clinic notes are less bulky but a glance at them will often reveal nothing more than a bewildering mass of sketchy hieroglyphics which are indecipherable to the non-ophthalmologist.

Medical records should accurately document:

1. The clinical findings at diagnosis.
2. The diagnosis and treatment.
3. The clinical findings at follow up and an indication of trends to allow an assessment of the effect of treatment and to prognosticate with a view to taking preventative action.
4. Changes in treatment and diagnosis during follow-up.

There are three types of data recorded during consultations for diabetic eye disease. They are:

1. Numerical data – e.g. date, distant visual acuity, near visual acuity, and intraocular pressure.
2. Pictorial: fundal appearances.
3. Narrative data.

Numerical data should not prove a problem. However, a sequential tabular record will allow a better appreciation of trends and provide easier access. An example is shown in *Table 7.6*. Here the data on right and left eyes is recorded in tabular fashion. Over a 9 month period from January to September the distant visual acuity on the right remained constant as did the near visual acuity and the intraocular pressure. However, on the left there was a progressive deterioration of visual acuity from 6/12 down to hand movements only. The intraocular pressure was high at the beginning of the year and although it was brought down with treatment no improvement in visual acuity was seen. These types of data are particularly amenable to computerization.

There are two forms of pictorial representation of fundal appearances.

The first involves the examiner making a sketch of fundal appearances on a previously prepared diagram. This can be in the form of a rubber stamp in the notes. This type of record is difficult to maintain

Table 7.6 Tabular record of numerical eye examination data

	Right			Left		
Date	*DVA*	*NVA*	*IOP*	*DVA*	*NVA*	*IOP*
2.1.86	6.09	5	21	6.12	0	30
6.5.86	6.09	5	20	6.60	0	28
11.9.86	6.09	5	18	0.02	0	21
		etc.			etc.	

accurately particularly when fundal changes become complex. It is almost impossible to quantify (See *Figure 7.4*).

The most accurate way of recording fundal appearances is by retinal photography. A series of colour photographs can be taken to cover the whole retina and be supplemented by fluoroscein

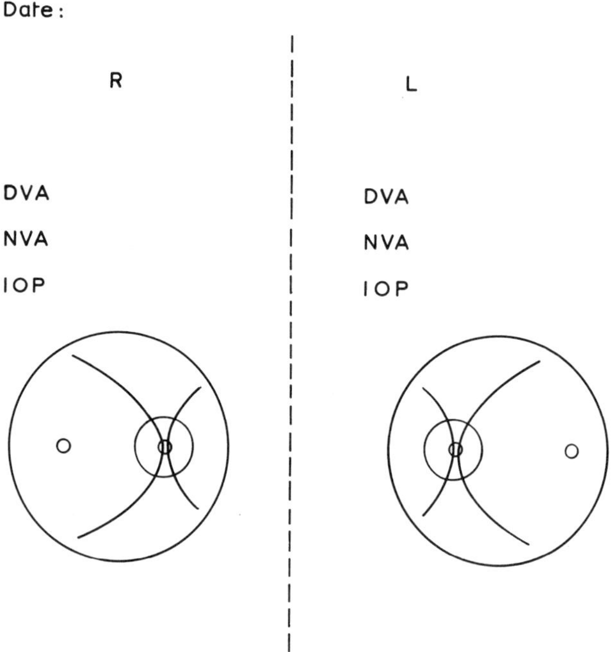

Figure 7.4 Pictorial representation of fundal appearance.

angiography. This, however, is expensive and time consuming and cannot be regarded as a method which could be adopted by the average diabetic clinic. In addition, if any form of analysis of these data is to take place the photographs need to be graded and converted to numerical data. This has been done at the Hammersmith Hospital, London, using the Hammersmith grading system. Although this has proved an excellent tool in the hands of experts, especially for research purposes, it is a non-starter for the average diabetic clinic.

Modern wide angle retinal cameras (e.g. CM3 – see screening for diabetic eye disease, and section 7.14) may provide an easy means of recording retinal appearances. Because of the wide angle fewer pictures need to be taken. However, again a numerical grading system is needed if any form of analysis and audit is to be undertaken.

Fundal appearances may be converted directly into numerical data at examination and recorded in the notes as such. This may be used by a diabetologist in secondary health care and by ophthalmic opticians and ophthalmic medical practitioners in primary health care. This system has the advantage that it has been tried and tested over a long period of time (14 years). It provides an adequate record of clinical data and the method has been found acceptable both in the diabetic clinic and for ophthalmic opticians working in primary health care.

The system involves three steps. The first is the acceptance of the definition of diabetic eye disease by those people working in the field. Secondly there must be acceptance of the documentation, and thirdly coding. *Table* 7.7 shows the diabetic eye disease record as completed in both primary and secondary health care. *Table 7.8* shows the coding used in the documentation. Although the coding may at first appear cumbersome it is rapidly learnt and the data quickly and easily recorded. The value of this type of documentation is that it forces the observer to note each of the retinal appearances in turn and make a decision about its severity. Actual appearances are recorded and not a diagnostic opinion as to the type of retinopathy present. This decision should be left to the expert managing the diabetic eye disease. This is preferably a diabetologist working in a Joint Retinal Clinic with an Ophthalmologist having a special interest in diabetic eye disease.

Table 7.7 Diabetic eye disease record as completed in both primary and secondary health care

Diabetic Eye Disease Programme		Observer................................
Surname		Hospital No. ....
Forename(s)		Date.....................................
	Notes	
	R. eye	L. eye
DVA	☐☐☐	☐☐☐
NVA	☐☐	☐☐
Cornea	☐	☐
Lens	☐	☐
Iris	☐	☐
Vitreous	☐	☐
IOP	☐☐	☐☐
Dots & blots	☐	☐
Hard exudates	☐	☐
Haemorrhage	☐	☐
Ischaemia	☐	☐
Proliferative retinopathy	☐	☐
Maculopathy	☐	☐
Medical treatment	☐	☐
Surgical treatment	☐☐☐☐	☐☐☐☐

DVA = Distant visual acuity with long distance spectacles (if worn) or pin hole.
NVA = Near visual acuity with reading spectacles (if worn).
IOP = Intraocular pressure.
For coding, see *Table 7.8*.

Table 7.8 Coding used for diabetic eye disease record in *Table 7.7*

DVA	000 = Blind 001 = Perception of light only 002 = Hand movements only 003 = Counting fingers at 1 metre Otherwise – record VA as 606 or 660 etc. (Snellen chart)

NAV	00 = Nil Otherwise – record as 05 etc. (round *up* to nearest whole number)
Cornea	0 = Normal 1 = Opacity 2 = Opacity preventing view of fundus
Lens	0 = Normal 1 = Opacity minimal with normal VA 2 = Opacity producing diminished VA 3 = Opacity preventing adequate view of fundus 4 = Cataract extraction
Iris	0 = Normal 1 = Rubeosis iridis 2 = Inadequate dil
Vitreous	0 = Normal 1 = Vitreous haemorrhage 2 = Vitreous haemorrhage preventing adequate view of fundus 3 = Asteroid hyalitis
IOP	Record pressure
Dots and blots	0 = Absent 1 = 1–2 present 2 = 3 or more 3 = Dot and blot threatening macula★
Hard exudates	0 = Absent 1 = Present but less than area of disc 2 = Present but greater than area of disc 3 = (not used) 4 = 1 'threatening macula'★ 5 = 2 'threatening macula'★
Haemorrhages	0 = Nil 1 = 1–2 present 2 = More than 2 present 3 = Not used 4 = 1–2 present 'threatening macula'★ 5 = More than 2 present 'threatening macula'★

★ Threatening the macula = lesion within the area of a circle centred on the fovea having a diameter equal to that of half the optic disc.

Retinal ischaemia	0 = Nil 1 = Definite (retinal infarcts 1–2 present) 2 = Definite (retinal infarcts 3 or more present) 3 = Suspected ischaemia: One or more of the following factors present Deep dark round haemorrhages Sheet haemorrhages Venous tortuosity or and/or dilatation IRMA (intra retinal microvascular abnormalities
Proliferative retinopathy	0 = No new vessels 1 = Peripheral new vessels only (PNV) 2 = Disc new vessels only (DNV) 3 = Retinitis proliferans (new vessels with fibrous proliferation 4 = PNV + DNV
Maculopathy	0 = Nil 1 = Exudative maculopathy 2 = Ischaemic maculopathy 3 = Non diabetic maculopathy
Medical treatment	0 = Nil 5 = Treatment for glaucoma
Surgical treatment	0000 = Nil, photocoagulation – record number of burns

The numerical data recorded in the Poole system is stored in a computer which allows ease of access and analysis of the data stored. (Clinical Data Systems, 41B King Street, Belper, Derbyshire, DE5 1PX).

Even without a computer the system provides a disciplined way of storing data recorded at the diabetic eye examination, whether it be during screening for diabetic eye disease, the initial secondary health care consultation, or in the diabetic eye disease follow up consultation.

There must always be a space in the notes for narrative data which cannot be converted into numerical data or reduced to coding.

7.12 THE PREVENTION AND TREATMENT OF DIABETIC RETINOPATHY

7.12.1 Prevention

Most diabetologists now believe that hyperglycaemia plays a major role in the causation of diabetic retinopathy. Various studies have been reported relating glycaemic control to the prevalence of retinopathy. Pirart (Pirart *et al.*, 1978) reported a series of 4000 patients observed over a period of 25 years. He showed that in those patients with the best control the prevalence of retinopathy was 20% compared with 80% for those with poor control and 40% for those with intermediately good control. Many other studies have also been done and all can be criticised on one count or another. Hyperglycaemia is now accepted as a major factor in the development of diabetic retinopathy and it is unlikely that a definitive double-blind control clinical trial will ever be done on good control versus bad control. It would now be unethical to carry out such a trial and in any case the trial would have to last many years before a definitie answer could be found. Animal studies should not be extrapolated to human experience except with great care. However, in one study it was shown that diabetic dogs with poor control developed retinopathy whereas diabetic dogs with good control did not (Engerman *et al.*, 1977).

It follows that in order to prevent the development of diabetic retinopathy it is essential to detect the diabetic in an early stage of his disease and then to follow him up at regular intervals to ensure that he maintains good glycaemic control in terms of home blood glucose monitoring, laboratory blood glucose monitoring, and HbA1 levels.

General measures such as blood pressure control, anti-smoking education, the lowering of blood lipids, and an awareness of the possible dangers of the contraceptive pill or pregnancy, should also be taken into account.

7.12.2 Treatment

The effect of good glycaemic control on established retinopathy is variable. Good glycaemic control is sometimes associated with regression but at other times with progression. In one study only near-normal glycaemia produced a slowing of the rate of formation of microaneurysms, haemorrhages and new vessels. There is also some evidence that tight diabetic control in certain situations may in fact accelerate the development of diabetic retinopathy. The cause for this is unknown but it may be that the retina has reached a point of no return and that at this point no matter what is done to blood glucose levels no improvement can be expected in the retina (Kohner *et al.*, 1982).

Other medications have been tried in diabetic retinopathy and found to have little effect. Vitamin B_{12} is of no value. A lipid lowering diet and lipid lowering agent do appear to reduce the number of hard exudates in the retina. However, they do not reduce the amount of retinal oedema and therefore have no effect on visual acuity. The antiplatelet properties of aspirin and dipyridamole have also been investigated but do not appear to affect the course of diabetic retinopathy.

Patients with established retinopathy should be followed up at regular intervals in order to ensure good glycaemic control, control of hypertension and normal serum lipids. They should be discouraged from smoking.

Any patient having the following indications should be seen by an ophthalmologist for confirmation of diagnosis and photocoagulation where indicated. It is in this situation that the value of joint retinal clinics run by an ophthalmologist and diabetologist is seen. A waiting time of less than 7 days can be achieved.

Indications for urgent referral to an ophthalmologist:

1. Neovascularization (DNV or PNV).
2. Preproliferative retinopathy.
3. Exudative retinopathy threatening the macula.
4. Maculopathy (ischaemic or exudative).

7.12.3 Photocoagulation

A high-energy beam of photons is directed onto the retina. The energy of the photons is absorbed and converted into thermal energy. This heat coagulates the surrounding area. The energy absorbed depends on the wavelength of the light used and on the intensity of the spot. It also depends upon the size of the spot.

Two sources are used for the high-energy beam of photons.

Non-coherent white light is produced by the xenon arc which is absorbed by the pigmented epithelium. This produces a full-thickness burn and cannot be used close to the fovea. Lasers (monochromatic coherent light) produce an intense beam of light which can be focused to a small area. The argon laser produces a wavelength of light which is absorbed well by the pigmented epithelium and is also absorbed by the haemoglobin in blood vessels. Photocoagulation beams directed at the pigmented epithelium produce a localized burn confined to the pigmented epithelium and the photoreceptor layer.

Photocoagulation is applied in two ways. Focal areas of the retina may be coagulated (focal photocoagulation – FPC) or large areas of the peripheral retina may be ablated (pan-photocoagulation – PPC). FPC may be used to destroy localized areas of leaking or new vessels but PPC is used to ablate large areas of peripheral retina which are still alive but ischaemic. This appears to reduce the stimulus to new vessel growth and disc new vessels then regress without local treatment.

7.12.4 Indications of photocoagulation

1. Disc new vessels – pan retinal photocoagulation.
2. Peripheral new vessels – pan photocoagulation or focal photocoagulation.
3. Maculopathy – focal photocoagulation.
4. Threatened maculopathy – focal photocoagulation.

It is important to treat threatened maculopathy before there is a deterioration in visual acuity since visual acuity lost through maculopathy cannot be recovered.

The successful application of photocoagulation in diabetic eye disease has reduced the incidence of blindness in threatened eyes by 60%.

7.13 ORGANIZATION OF THE DIABETIC EYE SERVICE

Like the general medical and surgical services the eye service may be divided into primary and secondary health care. In secondary health care Eye Departments and Eye Hospitals are serviced by consultant ophthalmologists and medical ophthalmologists. In the UK medical ophthalmologists are few and far between. Consultant ophthalmic surgeons have a long and arduous training. They are highly skilled and highly qualified. They are generally overworked and their waiting lists are long. It is unlikely that consultant ophthalmologists would be able to undertake routine screening for diabetic eye disease, nor should they be asked to do so.

In primary health care the family doctor may be the first member of the medical team to be consulted about eye problems. However, in the UK the majority of family doctors have little experience in the management of eye disease and are know to be unsure about their ability to screen effectively for diabetic eye disease. It is unlikely that a single practitioner would gain sufficient clinical experience to become efficient in this sphere.

Ophthalmic opticians (optomotrists) are not medically qualified. However, they have a University education and obtain a qualifying degree which in UK law allows them to undertake diagnostic examinations and to prescribe spectacles. It has been shown that they are able to screen effectively and efficiently for diabetic eye disease (Hill, 1981; Burns-Cox and Dean Hart, 1985).

Dispensing opticians dispense spectacles but may not prescribe them or carry out diagnostic examinations. However, some dispensing opticians do employ either ophthalmic opticians or ophthalmic medical practitioners (medical practitioners with eye training) who are able to undertake diagnostic examination and prescribe spectacles.

Ophthalmic medical practitioners are ideally suited to screen for diabetic eye disease. They are both medically trained and have a special training in ophthalmology.

The diabetologist must ensure that he has some training in medical ophthalmology. This is best obtained by working in a joint retinal clinic with a consultant ophthalmic surgeon

7.13.1 Screening

It has been suggested that there should be diabetic eye centres where patients would have an annual examination by an ophthalmologist after dilation of the pupil (Black and Bloom, 1978). This is not a practical proposition and indeed would be a gross misuse of the highly trained and highly skilled ophthalmologist. It is better that such skills should be devoted to the task of treating eye disease and solving diagnostic problems.

If it is considered that the whole of the diabetic population should have an annual eye examination (Foulds *et al.*, 1983), who should do the screening? This represents a considerable work load for the eye service. Even if it were appropriate for a specialist ophthalmologist to do screening it would be necessary to appoint many more ophthalmologists to cope with the work. Certainly there are not enough medical ophthalmologists to deal with this type of screening and it would be impossible to screen such a large number of patients within the diabetic clinic. In any case 50% of the patients are not attending diabetic clinics in the UK and any screening program confined to diabetic clinics would therefore miss 50% of the patients. Family doctors are unlikely to provide an effective screening program. Two other alternatives must be considered.

(a) Non-mydriatic retinal camera based screening program

This system uses a camera capable of taking a single wide-angle (45°) picture of the retina. It is able to do this without dilation of the pupil and gives a picture covering an area of the retina which extends from the disc to the macula and beyond. This is said to detect over 90% of lesions at the posterior pole. However, some peripheral lesions may be missed. The picture quality is good and a permanent polaroid record is obtained for the notes (Ryder *et al.*, 1982, 1984).

The advantages of this sytem are:

1. No mydriatic is used.
2. Only one photograph is taken and the examination is extremely rapid.
3. A permanent record is obtained for the notes.

The disadvantages of the system are as follows:

1. The patient may have to travel a considerable distance to where the camera is housed.
2. A camera must be provided, and housed. A receptionist and nurses must be available to organize the clinic.
3. A photographer (whether it be a trained photographer or trained other person) is necessary.

4. The photographs must be read after they have been taken by an experienced interpreter.
5. The visual acuity is not measured.
6. The intraocular pressure is not measured.
7. Errors of refraction are not corrected.
8. The capital outlay is expensive (see section 9.14).

(b) Ophthalmic optician (optomotrist) based screening program

In this system diabetic patients are given a list of ophthalmic opticians taking part in the diabetic eye disease screening program and are asked to attend for an annual examination. (Hill, 1981; Burns-Cox and Dean Hart, 1985). The system has the following advantages:

1. Patients are usually able to find an ophthalmic optician near to their home.
2. Because of the number of ophthalmic opticians involved the workload for any one ophthalmic optician is small.
3. The distant and near visual acuities are measured and refractory errors corrected. Spectacles may be prescribed if necessary.
4. Intraocular pressure is measured.
5. The pupils are dilated and a good view of the retina including the periphery is obtained.
6. By using a central reporting system it is possible to audit follow-up.

The system has the following disadvantages:

1. Because there are a large number of observers the errors of observation may be correspondingly large. However, this has been shown not to be the case (Hill, 1981).
2. Patients do have their eyes dilated.
3. It has been suggested that this system is very expensive (Waugh, 1986) (section 9.14 – Costs).

Having established an annual screening program provision must be made for further investigation of those found to have diabetic retinopathy. This is first-stage review; 26% of those screened will have retinopathy.

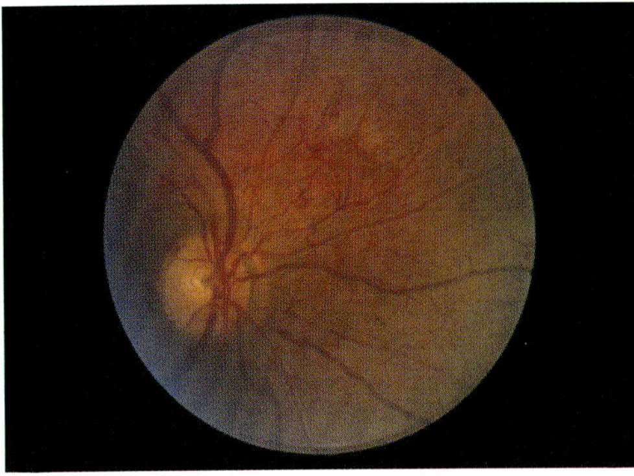

Plate 13 Proliferative retinopathy with peripheral new vessels. Patient aged 50 years, insulin-dependent diabetes for 20 years. Hypertensive. Photograph shows a fine leash of new vessels surrounding an area of ischaemic retina.

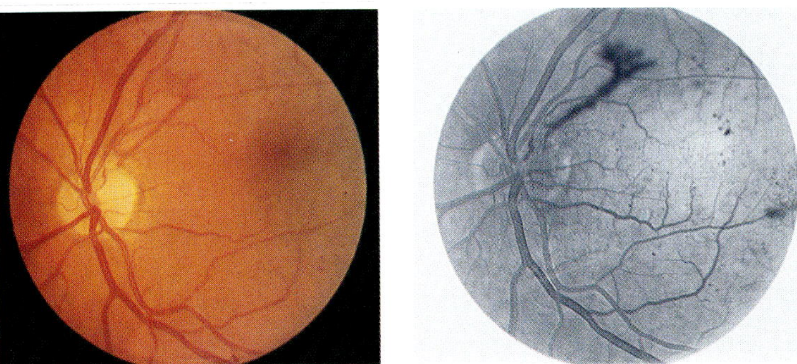

Plate 14 Proliferative retinopathy with disc new vessels. Patient aged 30 years, insulin-dependent diabetes for 20 years. Photograph shows abnormal leash of new vessels extending forward into the vitreous (and thus blurred on the colour photograph). The fluorescein angiograms show abnormal vessels leaking fluorescein.

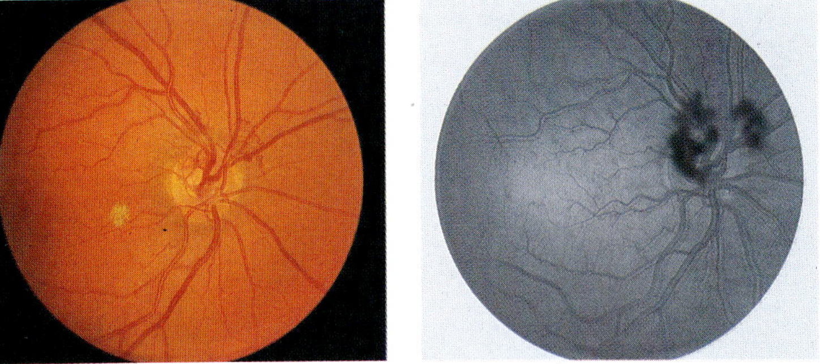

Plate 15 Proliferative retinopathy with disc new vessels. An apparently normal retina but with an area of new vessels arising from the disc. The nature of these vessels is clearly shown on the fluorescein angiogram. Fluorescein leaks from the abnormal vessels but does not leak from the normal retinal vessels.

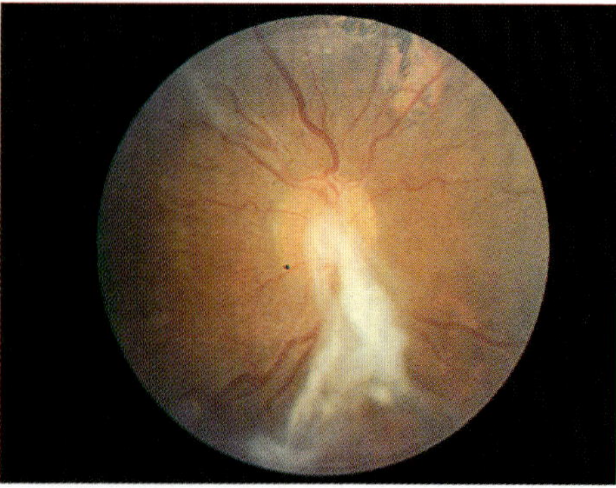

Plate 16 Retinitis proliferans. Patient aged 25 years, insulin-dependent diabetes for 20 years. Patient never accepted diabetes and refused to attend any clinic. During childhood required psychiatric treatment. Refused to attend adult diabetic clinic and completely neglected diabetes. Patient presented with severe symmetrical peripheral neuropathy and autonomic neuropathy giving rise to diabetic foot disease. Amputation of the right great toe required (Plate 23). Severe retinitis proliferans with a visual acuity of 6/18 in both eyes discovered during his admission.

Photograph shows extensive proliferation of fibrous tissue in a leash of new vessels arising from the disc.

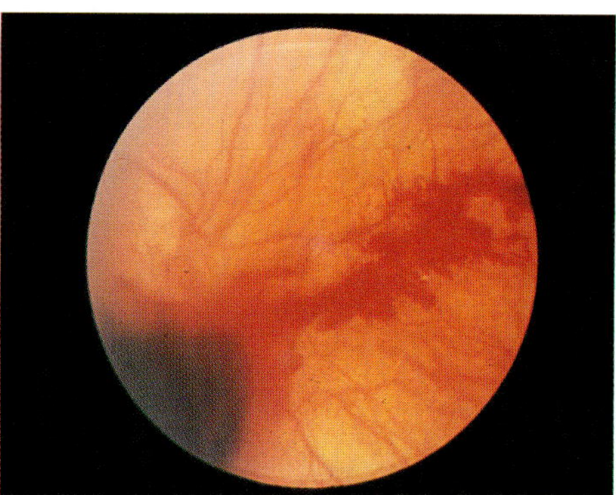

Plate 17 Vitreous haemorrhage from disc new vessels.

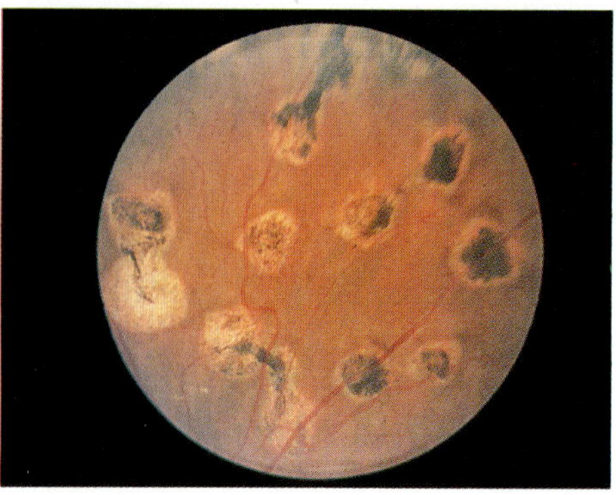

Plate 18 Photocoagulation burns.

Plate 19 Venous dilatation of autonomic neuropathy. Patient aged 45 years, duration of diabetes 20 years. Dilated veins on the dorsum of the foot associated with bounding peripheral pulses suggested autonomic neuropathy. A venous sample of blood was shown to be arterialized. Absent beat to beat variation, a raised vibration threshold at the ankle and diminished pin prick sensation over both feet completed the neuropathic picture.

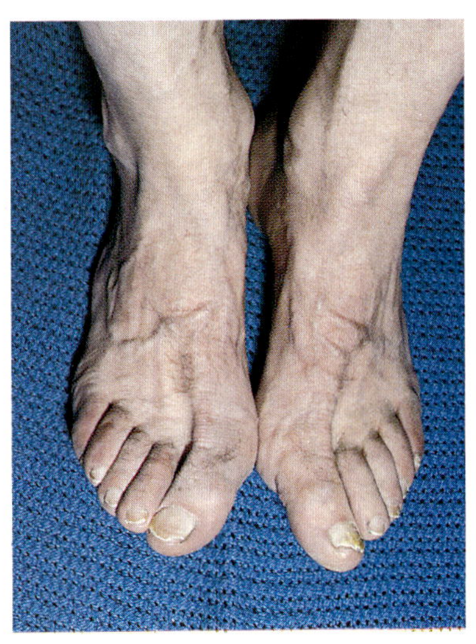

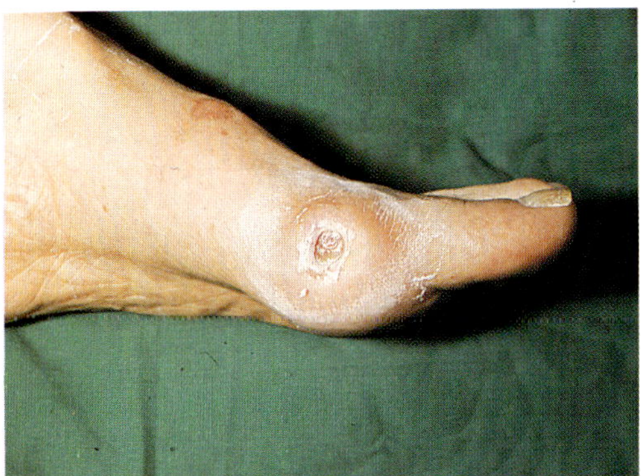

Plate 20 Neuropathic ulceration. Known duration of non-insulin dependent diabetes 5 years.

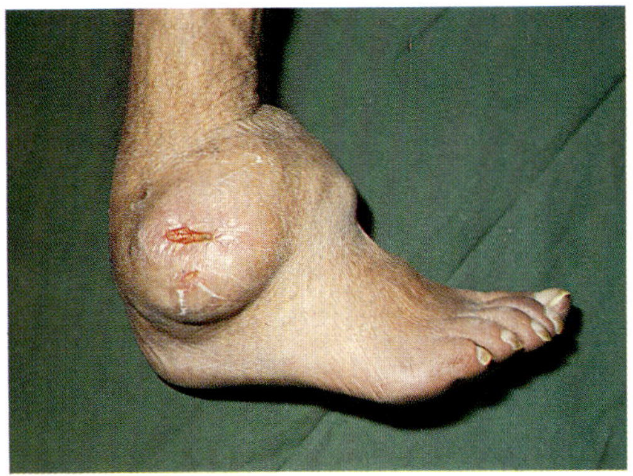

Plate 21 Charcot joint.

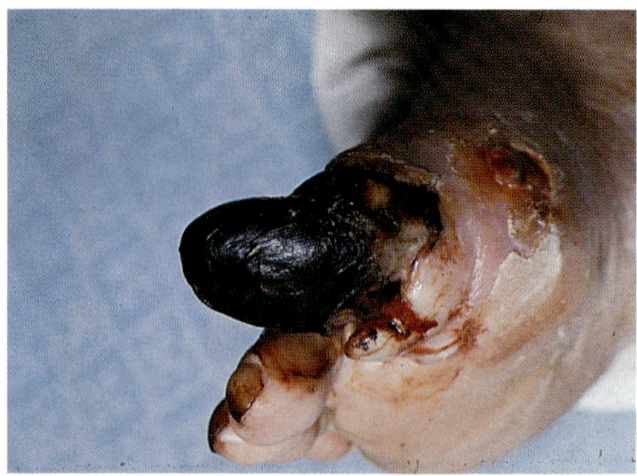

Plate 22 Ischaemic gangrene of the great toe. Male aged 50 years, duration of diabetes 5 years. Smoked 30 cigarettes per day since the age of 20. Two years previously complained of intermittent claudication with a claudicating distance of 100 yards. Developed ischaemic right great toe over a period of one month requiring amputation.

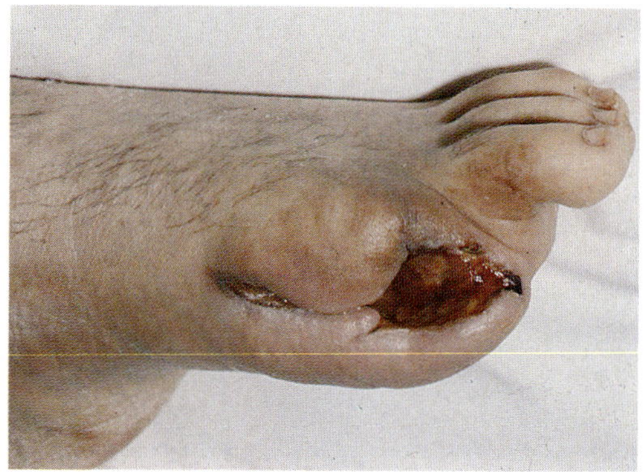

Plate 23 Neuropathic ulceration of the great toe associated with infection and leading to amputation. Same patient as referred to in Plate 16.

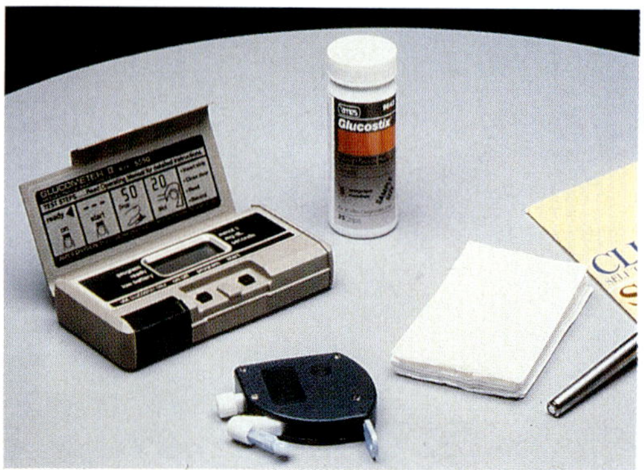

Plate 24 The Ames glucometer.

7.13.2 Who should perform first-stage review?

Primary health care does not contain the expertise necessary for first-stage review. This should be performed in secondary health care. The patients should not be referred to specialist ophthalmologists for first-stage review as this would unduly overload the specialist with a large proportion of cases with simple background retinopathy which do not require this level of expertise. However, it is essential that an expert assessment of the retina should be made and it is suggested that the diabetologist should take on this role. The training required is best obtained by working with an ophthalmologist in a joint retinal clinic. However, the first stage review should not be done in the joint retinal clinic but should be done in a separate clinic where a review of the patient as a whole may be made. In this clinic the following should be undertaken:

1. Check the findings of the eye disease screening program.
2. A review of risk factors.
3. A full assessment for the presence of other long-term complications.
4. Appropriate action taken on the findings.

Patients with confirmed retinopathy may be divided into four groups:

Group 1 – Those patients requiring urgent photocoagulation. These patients include those with new vessels and established maculopathy.

Group 2 – Patients requiring urgent follow-up by ophthalmologists, preferably in conjunction with a diabetologist at a joint retinal clinic. These patients include those with pre-proliferative retinopathy, and threatened maculopathy.

Group 3 – This includes patients who are a diagnostic problem and require referral to an ophthalmologist (preferably in a joint retinal clinic) for a diagnostic opinion.

Group 4 – Those patients with background retinopathy not threatening the macula and not pre-proliferative. This group of patients needs follow-up in the diabetic clinic setting for close supervision and regular assessment of the retinopathy to detect any progression.

7.13.3 Frequency of follow-up

The diabetic population should be screened on an annual basis. Group 4 patients above should be reviewed by the diabetologist on a six monthly basis or more frequently if he thinks this is necessary. Group 3 patients should be recategorized in the light of the ophthalmologist's opinion. Groups 1 and 2 patients should be followed up at 3 monthly intervals or at intervals determined necessary by the ophthalmologist following photocoagulation.

7.13.4 Time scale

Lines of communication must be established between those effecting the screening program and the point of first stage review. For urgent cases (e.g. Group 1 and Group 2 above) there should be no delay between screening and referral.

Those patients requiring urgent photocoagulation (Group 1 above) should be seen by an ophthalmologist within two weeks of first stage review.

Those patients in Groups 2 and 3 should be seen by the specialist ophthalmologist within 2–4 weeks of first stage review depending on the urgency determined by the diabetologist.

It may be considered that the scheme of action outlined above is impossible to achieve in practice. This may be the case in areas without efficient co-operation between primary health care (particularly ophthalmic opticians), the ophthalmologist, and the diabetologist; however the following time scale has been achieved in the Community Care Service, for Diabetics in the Poole Area:

1. Screen to central report – 1 week or less.
2. Central report to stage one review – 1 week or less.
3. Stage one review to stage two review/follow-up:
   (i) Group 1 – 2 weeks or less.
   (ii) Groups 2/3 – 4 weeks or less.
   (iii) Group 4 – 3–6 month intervals.
4. Urgency determined at:
   (i) Screening session.
   (ii) Central reporting session.
   (iii) Stage 1 review.

By defining areas of responsibility within the primary and secondary health care sections of the service it has been possible to exploit expertise to the full. This has meant that the skills and experience of the ophthalmologists are not wasted on screening programmes or even first review but can be exploited to the full to provide necessary diagnostic second opinions and treatment. The division of responsibility between screening, first review and second review, has speeded up communication and reduced waiting times.

7.14 COSTS

The costs in a diabetic screening programme are considered in this section. A comparison is made between the costs in annual screening of all diabetics by an ophthalmic optician based system compared with a camera based system. In order to make a comparison a population unit of 100 000 will be considered. This would expect to yield 1000 diabetics. We may therefore consider the costs of an annual screening programme for 1000 diabetics.

7.14.1 Ophthalmic optician based system

At 1986 prices the screening of an individual patient for diabetic eye disease, including the usual clinical examination involved on consultation of an ophthalmic optician, is £8.50. The cost involved is therefore £8500 per annum per unit population.

7.14.2 Camera based system

It has been reported that the screening (1 photograph of each eye) of a patient by this method takes 6 minutes. We may therefore assume that 6000 minutes per annum will be required to screen 1000 patients. Allowing for a 3 hour session (180 minutes) this would indicate that 33 sessions would be required as a minimum to screen 1000 patients.

The costs may be approximated as follows:

1. Camera (Cannon CR3 – 45 NM) approximately £11 000. If the camera life is approximately 8 years this would involve a cost per annum of £1440
2. Film at £1.50 per person 1500
3. Operator, 33 sessions per annum 685

4. Receptionist	685
5. Nurse	685
6. Hidden costs – rent, light, heat, medical records, secretary	?
Total minimum	£5000 p.a. +

The cost is thus at least £5000 p.a. per unit population.

7.14.3 Comment

It would appear from the above estimates that screening by ophthalmic opticians is almost twice as expensive as screening by the camera method. This of course assumes that the camera continues to operate for 8 years and there are no breakdowns and no maintenance is required. However, all is not what it seems.

The two methods of screening are not comparable. Ophthalmic opticians measure visual acuity and if necessary correct refractive errors and can prescribe spectacles. The camera method of screening does not do this. In addition ophthalmic opticians measure intraocular pressure and there is thus built into the screening programme a screen for glaucoma. The camera method does not have this provision. Using ophthalmic opticians for screening should prevent loss of vision from glaucoma in this group of patients.

The camera method may be more convenient as the patient does not require dilated pupils for the examination, but on the other hand periperal lesions will be missed. Patients have to travel to where the camera is situated. Most patients can find an ophthalmic optician working close to home.

There are also other factors relating to cost; 26% of patients will be found to have retinopathy after the initial screening programme and will be followed up elsewhere. In addition, a large proportion of patients are already attending ophthalmic opticians. In one survey, 71% had attended an ophthalmic optician within the preceding 2 years and 52% within the preceding year; 69% were currently wearing spectacles (Burns-Cox and Dean Hart, 1986). These factors must significantly reduce the estimated cost of a screening programme based on ophthalmic opticians.

It also must be remembered that the ophthalmic optician provides his own consulting room with all ancillary staff. A camera used for screening must be housed in suitable accommodation with hidden costs of heating, lighting and servicing.

All these factors must be taken into account when deciding how to screen for diabetic retinopathy. Whatever the method chosen and the ultimate cost it should be set against the actual savings which would accrue from preventing blindness (annual cost £3500 for each case of blind registration (Foulds, 1983)).

7.15 A SUGGESTED PLAN OF ACTION

A summary of a plan of action is as follows:

1. Register ALL diabetics in area.
2. Organize screening programme. Ophthalmic optician/camera based.
3. Inform all patients and doctors of the existence of this programme. Individual letters, personally addressed asking all patients to attend for annual screen.
4. Screening programme : organized recall (annual) (word processor).
5. Organize central reporting session – to deal with screening reports (e.g. letters, ophthalmic optician reports, Polaroid pictures, etc.).
6. Organize first-stage review session.
7. Organize second-stage review session:
   (i) Preferably with joint retinal clinic (diabetologist and ophthalmic surgeon).
   (ii) Diabetic clinic with special facilities.

There should not be more than 1 week's delay between the screen and a review of the result centrally. Similarly there should not be more than 2 weeks' delay between the receipt of the report and stage-1 review. The waiting time between stage 1 and stage 2 review will depend on the urgency as indicated by the grouping of patients. At each stage of the programme the urgency will be determined on an individual basis.

To achieve this level of efficiency it is essential to have an organized system of care.

It is essential to register all diabetics within the area. This includes those (up to 50%) who do not attend the diabetic clinic and may be receiving indifferent care from their local doctors. The register may be compiled from a register of patients attending the diabetic clinic, family doctor practice disease registers, repeat prescriptions, and by making family doctors and receptionists aware of the need to include everybody on a register.

It is then necessary to organize a screening programme. This will obviously depend on local conditions and need. It may be centrally situated in a hospital, either ophthalmic optician based or non-mydriatic camera based, or community based (ophthalmic optician).

All patients on the diabetic register and doctors in the area should be informed of the existence of the diabetic eye disease programme. Individual letters, personally addressed, asking all patients to attend for an annual eye screen should be sent to all patients on the diabetic register. A word processor in this situation is invaluable.

Built into the screening programme, whether it is organized centrally or peripherally, should be an annual recall system.

Reports of the screening examination should be directed to a central address for reporting. One senior person should be responsible for looking at all reports and making decisions.

It is necessary to organize a first-stage review session and to decide how to deal with those patients who have retinopathy. A second-stage review session is important and it is preferable that this should be in the form of a joint retinal clinic with a diabetologist and ophthalmologist working together. The diabetic clinic for follow-up of routine patients not referred to the joint retinal clinic should have the facilities for examination of the eye.

During the first years of any diabetic eye disease programme the workload will be considerable because of the heavy back-log of previous undiscovered retinopathy. However, as time passes the situation will be controlled and the work load eased.

Perseverance and singleness of purpose is required here!

REFERENCES AND FURTHER READING

Black, R.K. and Bloom, A. (1978) Diabetic eye centres for the management of diabetic eye disease. *Health Trends*, **10**, 88–90.

Burns-Cox, C.J. and Dean Hart, J.C. (1985) Screening of diabetics for retinopathy by ophthalmic opticians. *Br. Med. J.*, **290**, 1052–54.

Burns-Cox, and Dean Hart, J.C. (1986) Advantages and costs of screening with non-mydriatic fundus camera. *Practical Diabetes*, **3**, 166.

Engerman, R., Bloodworth, J.M.B. and Nelson, S. (1977) Relationship of microvascular disease in diabetes to metabolic control. *Diabetes*, **26**, 760–69.

Foulds, W.S., MacCuish, A.C., Barrie, T., *et al.* (1983) Diabetic retinopathy in the West of Scotland: its detection and prevalence and the cost effectiveness of a proposed screening programme. *Health Bull. (Edin.)*, **41**, 318–26.

Hill, R.D. (1981) Primary health care screening programme for diabetic eye disease. *Diabetologia*, **20**, 670.

Kohner, E.M., McLeod, D. and Marshal, J. (1982) Complications of Diabetes. *Diabetic Eye Disease* (Ed. Keen and Jarrett), 2nd edn, Edward Arnold, London, Chapter 2.

Kritzinger, E.E. and Taylor, G. (1984) *Diabetic Eye Disease.* MTP Press, Lancaster.

Pirart, J., Lauvaux, J.P. and Rey, W. (1978) Blood sugar and diabetic complications (letter). *N. Engl. J. Med.*, **298**, 1149.

Ryder, R.E.J., Young, S., Vora, J., Atiea, J.A., Owens, D.R. and Hayes, T.M. (1985) Screening for diabetic retinopathy using polaroid retinal photography through undilated pupils. *Practical Diabetes*, **2(5)**, 34–40.

Ryder, R.E.J., Young, S., Hayes, T.M. and Owens, D.R. (1984) Canon CR2 – 45 NM retinal camera markedly improves detection of diabetic retinopathy through undilated pupils (Abstract No. 455). *Diabetologia*, **27**, 326A.

Waugh, N.R., Ellingford, A. and Scott, S.D. (1986) Screening for diabetic retinopathy: options and cost effectiveness. *Practical Diabetes,* **3(1)**, 30–1.

· Eight ·

Diabetic nephropathy

8.1 INTRODUCTION

The functional unit of the kidney is the nephron. This consists of a high-pressure filter (the glomerulus) and a complex renal tubular system.

The glomerulus consists of a knot of capillaries supplied by the afferent arteriole (derived from branches of the renal artery) and drained by the efferent arteriole. The filtration pressure within the glomerulus is dependent upon the vascular tone of the arterioles. The wall of the glomerulus acts as a filtration barrier. It effectively separates cells and large molecules from small molecules and water which pass through the filtration barrier to form the glomerular filtrate. The rate at which the filtrate is formed (the glomerular filtration rate or GFR) is a measure of renal function.

The filtration barrier is complex. The wall of the glomerular capillary consists of an inner lining of endothelial cells, the basement membrane and outer layer of covering epithelial cells. The rate at which the filtrate passes through the filtration barrier and the size of the molecule allowed to pass depends upon many factors. Of these the filtration pressure, the membrane charge, the charge on the molecules being filtered, and the structural integrity of the filtration barrier appear to be the most important. Changes in the function and structural integrity of the filtration barrier are reflected in the molecular constituents of the glomerular filtrate. A damaged 'leaky' glomerulus will allow the passage of larger molecules than normal. This forms the basis of further tests of renal function and in particular of the integrity of the filtration barrier. Under normal circumstances, because of its size, shape and charge, very little albumin appears in the glomerular filtrate and thus eventually in the urine. Measurement of the albumin excretion rate (AER) provides a useful measure of glomerular filtration barrier integrity.

After filtration, the glomerular filtrate passes into the complex renal tubular system. It passes through the proximal convoluted tubule, the loop of Henle, the distal convoluted tubule and eventually via the collecting ducts into the renal pelvis. During its passage crystalloids are removed from and added to the glomerular filtrate in order to maintain the internal milieu. The product arriving in the renal pelvis following the process of modification is urine. The concentration of substances in the urine thus depends on a complex process with many modifying factors. The concentration of glucose appearing in the urine depends not only upon the amount of glucose filtered (and therefore the blood glucose concentration) but also upon the amount of glucose reabsorbed from the glomerular filtrate as it passes down the renal tubular system. The capacity to reabsorb glucose varies from person to person. If more glucose is filtered than can be absorbed (i.e. the renal threshold for glucose is exceeded) then glucose appears in the urine. The actual concentration of glucose will also depend on the amount of water extracted from the glomerular filtrate. It will be seen that the measurement of concentrations of substances in the urine may not be a very accurate way of assessing either blood concentration or renal function. This is particularly so when the concentration and amounts of substances measured are very small. Actual excretion rates more accurately reflect nephron function. The problem with the measurement of excretion rates lies in the necessity for timed urine specimens, a notoriously difficult procedure to perform accurately. However, albumin excretion rates (AER) have been measured and compared in diabetics and in non-diabetics. The albumin excretion rate is thought to reflect the functional integrity of the filtration barrier.

8.1.1 Normoalbuminuria

Normal values of the albumin excretion rate depend on the precise method of measurement (24 hour urine, overnight urine, supine, erect, at rest, or with exercise). Mogensen has attempted to define very precisely the albumin excretion rate in non-diabetics under strictly defined conditions. An albumin excretion rate of 2.3–8.3 μg per minute or 3.3–11.9 mg per 24 hours is defined as normoalbuminuria. However, Viberti gives the upper limit of normal as twice this value. The confusion between albumin excretion rate and albumin concentration (AC) is considerable. The pundits confuse us further by sometimes expressing albuimin excretion rates (AER) in μg per minute or mg per 24 hours! For a given albumin excretion rate the concentration of albumin appearing in the urine will depend on how much water is present in the urine specimen. The concentration will fall in the presence of a diuresis and rise in the presence of dehydration. However, as the albumin excretion rate rises the albumin concentration increases and may then be detectable by simple measurement of albumin concentration (e.g. Albustix).

8.1.2 Macroalbuminuria

In the absence of infected urine, an intermittently positive Albustix test indicates intermittent macroalbuminuria. When the urine test becomes consistently positive the test indicates persistent macroalbuminuria. A positive Albustix test usually indicates an albumin excretion rate greater than 200–250 mg per 24 hours or 140–174 μg per minute. These terms must be distinguished from the term microalbuminuria which is defined on the basis of an albumin excretion rate.

8.1.3 Microalbuminuria

The albumin excretion rate which exceeds the normal range (and this depends on its definition!) but falls short of detection by simple tests of proteinuria (e.g. Albustix) is said to indicate microalbuminuria. *Table 8.1* gives useful working definitions of normoalbuminuria, microalbuminuria and macroalbuminuria. Whether an AER of 174 μg/min (250 mg/24 hours) is enough to make the Albustix test

Table 8.1 Albuminuria

		Albumin excretion rate	
	Albustix	*μg/min*	*mg/24 hours*
Normoalbuminuria	—	2.8–8.3	3.3–11.9
Microalbuminuria	—	18–174	26–250
Macroalbuminuria:			
intermittent	±	174	250
persistent	+	174	250

positive will depend entirely upon how concentrated the urine is (i.e. how much water has been extracted from the glomerular filtrate during its passage down the renal tubule).

8.1.4 The significance of microalbuminuria

Persistent macroalbuminuria is the prime indicator of diabetic nephropathy. Microalbuminuria is, however, very variable and the level at which the albumin excretion rate indicates significant disorder of the filtration barrier is the subject of much debate (AER 10–70 μg per minute or 14.4–100.8 mg per 24 hours). Viberti *et al.* (1982) and Jarrett *et al.* (1984) showed that an albumin excretion rate of 30 μg per minute or more was a good predictor of future renal failure in insulin-dependent diabetics and of mortality in non-insulin dependent diabetics.

By the time persistent macroalbuminuria is established the typical histological features of diabetic nephropathy are well advanced. The basement membrane of the glomerulus becomes thickened. The degree of thickening is a function of time and is thus related to the duration of diabetes. The diffuse thickening of the basement membrane is also associated with an increase in the basement membrane like material in the mesangium. Large clumps of this material accumulate and eventually light microscopic appearances of the Kimmelstiel–Wilson kidney appear (nodular glomerulosclerosis). There is thus a gradual and progressive destruction of the functioning nephons in the kidney which in some cases eventually leads to chronic renal failure.

The functional changes seen in diabetic nephropathy have been extensively studied. Initially, the glomerular filtration rate is increased and the kidneys are enlarged. As time progresses, in many cases there is a progressive fall in the glomerular filtration rate leading to the retention of creatinine and urea.

Abnormal renal function is also indicated by an increased leak of albumin into the urine. An abnormal albumin excretion rate is probably the earliest sign of glomerular malfunction in diabetes.

8.2 THE STAGES OF DIABETIC NEPHROPATHY

The natural history of diabetic nephropathy is the subject of considerable debate. It has, as yet, not been fully elucidated. However,

Mogensen has defined five stages in the natural history of diabetic renal disease affecting patients with insulin dependent diabetes (Mogensen, 1983).

This definition provides a useful working hypothesis.

8.2.1 Stage 1. Renal hyperfunction (hyperfiltration) and hypertrophy

This stage is symptomless. It occurs at diagnosis and on occasions when metabolic control is poor. This stage is characterized by a raised glomerular filtration rate, large kidneys and microalbuminuria. These features return to normal when good glycaemic control is attained and then maintained. Renal biopsy at this time shows a normal structure and no thickening of the glomerular basement membrane. If control is imperfect then elements of stage 1 remain.

8.2.2 Stage 2. Silent nephropathy

This stage is also symptomless. However, the glomerular filtration rate is increased as is kidney size. The albumin excretion rate may be normal but on exercise and during episodes of poor control it increases. The characteristic feature of this stage is glomerular basement membrane thickening.

8.2.3 Stage 3. Incipient nephropathy

This stage is also symptomless. It is characterized by microalbuminuria. Routine testing with Albustix is therefore negative. The presence of microalbuminuria (equal to or greater than 30 μg per min) predicts the development of overt clinical nephropathy during the next 10 years in a significant proportion of patients.

Patients with a glomerular filtration rate of less than 130 ml per minute may show little or no progression. Patients with hyperfiltration (a glomerular filtration rate of 150 ml per minute or more) have an increased risk of developing overt nephropathy.

The diastolic blood pressure is raised is this group (90 compared with 70–80 mm Hg in controls) though not to the usually accepted levels seen in hypertension. It is considered that this rise in blood pressure may be of renal origin. It may be a contributory factor in the development of clinical nephropathy since treatment of blood pressure slows progression.

The progression of patients from stage 2 to stage 4 is indicated by an increase in albumin excretion rate of 20% per annum. Eventually intermittent proteinuria with Albustix positivity becomes apparent (*Table 8.1*).

8.2.4 Stage 4. Overt diabetic nephropathy

This stage is also asymptomatic. The albumin excretion rate increases to around 200 μg per minute or more and persistent proteinuria (i.e. Albustix positive) is apparent. The blood pressure rises to hypertensive levels (i.e. 160/95 or more) and there is a linear fall of glomerular filtration rate of 1 ml per minute per month. The rate of progression is affected by poor metabolic control, blood pressure and high solute load.

8.2.5 Stage 5. End stage diabetic renal failure (chronic renal failure)

In this stage the patients become symptomatic. The glomerular filtration rate progressively falls and is usually accompanied by a fall in albumin excretion rate. The blood pressure rises and 66% of patients entering this stage, if untreated, die of uraemia and 33% die of coronary artery disease.

Non insulin dependent diabetics have not been observed to pass through stage 1. The hyperfiltration of stages 2 and 3 has not been demonstrated. However, very little is known about the natural history of diabetic renal failure in non insulin dependent diabetics.

8.3 SCREENING FOR DIABETIC RENAL DISEASE

All patients with diabetes should be initially and annually screened for nephropathy, as follows:

1. All patients – initial and annual screen:
   (i) Early morning urine : dipstick (Albustix) test for albumin.
   (ii) Serum creatinine.
   (iii) MSU for microscopy and culture.

2. Selected patients (see text):
   (i) EMU A/C ratio.
   (ii) Overnight AER.

Patients should be asked to supply an early morning urine (EMU – i.e. the urine passed on rising) for a simple Albustix test. A mid-stream speciment of urine (MSU) should be sent to the laboratory for microscopy and culture. The serum creatinine should be measured.

The ideal urine specimen for assessing the albumin excretion or albumin concentration (Albustix) is unknown and is the subject of discussion. (Gatling, Knight and Hill, 1984, 1985). The early morning urine (EMU) is advised since it is less affected by exercise and posture. In addition, the original work on albumin excretion rates in relation to the development of nephropathy was done using overnight collections of urine (Viberti *et al.*, 1982).

If the MSU indicates infection then this should be treated and the screening test repeated.

Insulin dependent diabetics under the age of 65 years whose EMU is not Albustix positive, and is not infected, should be investigated further. An aliquot of the EMU should be sent to the laboratory for an albumin/creatinine ratio (A/C ratio).

Although the albumin excretion rate would be a more definitive screening test, the problem of collecting timed urine specimens from a large number of patients should not be underestimated. In addition, the timing of urine collections is often inaccurate. To overcome the problem of variable urine concentration an alternative is to measure the urinary albumin concentration in mg/1 (A) and the urinary creatinine in mmol/1 (C). An A/C ratio of 3.5 or more is an indication for further investigation by measuring the albumin excretion rate.

This A/C ratio has a senstitivity of 100% with a predictive value of 64%. On this basis, only 13% of all patients tested will have an early morning urine albumin creatinine ratio of 3.5 or more and it will only be necessary for these patients to submit urine for an albumin excretion rate measurment (Gatling *et al.*, 1985). By measuring the A/C ratio large numbers of patients may be screened for microalbuminuria with the minimum of effort. It should not be forgotten that microalbuminuria is very variable and may be present on one occasion and not on another.

8.4 RENAL FOLLOW-UP

If any of the following are positive, further investigation and renal follow-up should be undertaken:

1. Albustix positive urine.
2. An albumin/creatinine ratio of 3.5 or more.
3. A serum creatine greater than 150 μmol/1 (1.7 mg%).

Other causes of abnormal renal function should be excluded and if necessary renal biopsy undertaken.

The tests necessary for renal follow-up in diabetic nephropathy are as follows:

1. AER (overnight).
2. Biochemistry:
   (i) Serum creatinine.
   (ii) Electrolytes.
   (iii) Urea.
   (iv) Albumin.
   (v) Urate.
   (vi) Blood glucose (IBS).
3. Haematology:
   (i) HbA1.
   (ii) Haemoglobin.
4. GFR (Cr. EDTA).
5. MSU (Microscopy and culture).
6. Blood pressure (lying and standing).

These should be performed at 3–6 month intervals. An albumin excretion rate (AER) should be measured on an overnight collection of urine. The glomerular filtration rate (GFR) should be estimated using the Cr. EDTA method. A midstream specimen of urine (MSU) should be sent to the laboratory for microscopy and culture. The blood pressure both lying and standing should be measured after a 10 minute rest. Glycaemic control should be assessed in terms of home blood glucose monitoring, interval blood sugar and HbA1. Other biochemical parameters should be measured as indicated.

The 3–6 monthly assessment will define the following:

1. The stage of renal involvement.
2. The rate of progression in terms of albumin excretion rate and renal impairment.

3. Blood pressure.
4. Infection.

The definition of the above parameters will enable therapeutic measures to be aimed at slowing the decline of renal function.

8.5 THERAPEUTIC MEASURES AIMED AT SLOWING THE DECLINE OF RENAL FUNCTION

The following therapeutic measures are available:

1. Good glycaemic control.
2. Blood pressure control (Mogenson, 1985).
3. Decrease in solute load (*Table 8.2*).
4. Treat genitourinary tract infection.

Good glycaemic control is valuable. Home blood glucose monitoring with preprandial blood glucose levels between 3–7 mmol/1 should be the aim. Similarly, the interval blood sugar as measured in the laboratory should be between 3 and 7 mmol/1 and at worst not greater than 10 mmol/1. The HbA1 should be within normal limits. However, it must be remembered that HbA1 values may not reflect glycaemic control accurately in the presence of renal failure, suggesting better glycaemic control than actually exists.

The blood pressure should be maintained at levels of 130–140 systolic and 85–90 diastolic. The blood pressure is probably best treated with a calcium antagonist (e.g. nifedipine) or ACE inhibitor (e.g. enalapril). Thiazide diuretics tend to worsen diabetic control and raise the serum urate. Beta blockers may be used in conjunction with a calcium antagonist or ACE inhibitor. A cardioselective beta blocker such as atenolol should be used initially at the dose of 50 mg daily. Beta blockers may effect the peripheral circulation increasing the danger of tissue necrosis if the limb is already at risk from arteriosclerosis.

A decrease in solute load has been shown to slow the decline in renal function. This may be achieved by decreasing protein intake. The protein actually eaten must be first class protein. *Table 8.2* indicates suitable quantities of protein to be taken in relation to the serum creatinine concentration. Due allowance for urinary protein loss must be made in the nephrotic syndrome.

Table 8.2 Decreasing the solute load. First class protein intake in relation to serum creatinine concentration

Serum creatinine		*Protein intake*
mmol/l	*mg%*	*g/day*
Less than 300	3.39	1–1.25 g/kg body weight
300–400	3.39–4.52	40–50 g/day

The serial measurement of parameters at 3–6 monthly intervals will demonstrate the efficiency of the above therapeutic measures and at the same time give a good indication of the rate of decline in renal function. Although rates of decline are very variable, for an individual patient, the decline is often linear, particularly in the later stages of the disease. This enables planned management of patients passing through the various stages of diabetic renal disease to chronic renal failure.

8.6 MANAGEMENT OF CHRONIC RENAL FAILURE

Only 5–7 years may elapse between the time the patient develops persistent proteinuria to the development of end stage chronic renal failure. Once the serum creatinine level has reached 200 μmol/1 or more there is often a linear fall in renal function and death from end stage renal failure may be expected in two years if untreated. It is only by detection of the at risk diabetic in the early stages of renal involvement that this progression can be slowed. A patient may be regarded as having entered the stage of chronic renal failure when the serum creatinine is 150 μmol/1 (1.7 mg%) or more.

The patient with chronic renal failure is likely to have other problems related to diabetes. The patient must be treated as a whole since many factors are interrelated and will affect one another. Patients in this group are likely to be hypertensive, have angina pectoris, cerebrovascular disease, peripheral vascular disease, retinopathy and neuropathy. In addition, glycaemic control may be poor and genitourinary tract infections may be present. During this stage the diabetologist should attempt to maintain good glycaemic control, treat hyperuricaemia, hyperlipidaemia, hypertension and genitourinary tract infections.

An all-out attempt should be made to treat these various conditions to obtain an optimal state. If this is done then the patient's well being will be vastly improved.

Diabetics in chronic renal failure require intensive follow-up. They need to be seen at 1–3 monthly intervals. A joint renal/diabetic clinic is ideal.

At the follow-up clinic the weight should be measured and the patient examined for a raised JVP, oedema, and basal crackles as an indication of fluid overload. Pulse, blood pressure (lying and standing) should be measured to monitor hypotensive therapy and to detect postural hypotension. Retinopathy may progress rapidly in chronic renal failure and it is essential to examine the retina at regular intervals and refer to an ophthalmologist for photocoagulation if necessary.

The serum creatinine, blood urea, electrolytes, calcium, phosphate, urate, alkaline phosphatase, and serum albumin should be measured. Glycaemic control should be assessed on the basis of the patient's own home blood glucose monitoring, the 2 hour interval blood glucose measured in the laboratory, and the haemoglobin A1. The total haemoglobin should be measured.

As a further assessment of hypertensive control the ECG and chest X-ray should be taken. In preparation for transplantation tissue typing and hepatitis antigens should be measured.

Early referral to a renal physician is essential. Patients should be referred when the creatinine has reached 300 μmol/1 (3.39 mg%). Diabetics should be taken into the end stage renal failure programme when the serum creatinine reaches 500 μmol/1 (5.6 mg%) (compared with non-diabetics when the serum creatinine is 800–1000 μmol/1, 9.0–11.3 mg%). Early entry into the End Stage Renal Failure Programme has dramatically improved the results for patients with end stage diabetic renal disease. Early continuous ambulatory peritoneal dialysis (CAPD) should be the aim although early transplant is even better.

8.7 CONCLUSION

Chronic renal failure is unpleasant and distressing for the patient. Gentle education, explanation, reassurance and support is at all times essential. This must not be forgotten in a busy clinic and fascination with metabolites should not obscure the physician's duty to treat the patient as a whole person and not a metabolic disorder.

REFERENCES AND FURTHER READING

Gatling, W., Knight, C. and Hill, R.D. (1984, 1985) Screening for diabetic nephropathy: Which urine sample? *Diabetologia* (1984), **27**, 277–78 (abstract). *Diab. Med* (1985), **2**, 451–55.

Keen, H. and Jarrett, R.J. (eds) (1982) *Complications of Diabetes*, 2nd edn. Edward Arnold, London.

Jarrett, R.J. Viberti, G.C., Argyropoulos, A., Hill, R.D., Mahmud, U., and Murrells, T.J. (1984) Microalbuminuria predicts mortality in non-insulin dependent diabetes. *Diab. Med.*, **1**, 17.

Mogensen, C.E., Christensen, C.K. and Vittinghus, E. (1983) The stages in diabetic renal disease with emphasis on the stage of incipient diabetic nephropathy. *Diabetes*, **32**, (Suppl. 2), 64–78.

Mogensen, C.E. (1984) Microalbuminuria and incipient diabetic nephropathy. *Diabetic Nephropathy*, **3**, 75.

Mogensen, C.E. (1985) Hypertension and Diabetes. *Practical Diabetes*, Vol. 2, **4**, 8–14.

Viberti, G.C., Hill, R.D., Jarrett, R.J., Argyropoulos, A., Mahmud, U. and Keen, H. (1982) Microalbuminuria as a predictor of clinical nephropathy in insulin dependent diabetes mellitus. *Lancet*, **1(i)**, 1430–32.

· Nine ·

Macrovascular disease

9.1 INTRODUCTION

Large vessel disease (atherosclerosis/arteriosclerosis) appears to occur as a natural consequence of the ageing process. Certain risk factors have been identified which increase the chances of developing macrovascular disease. These are as follows:

1. Age.
2. Smoking.
3. Hypertension.
4. Diabetes.
5. Hyperlipidaemia.
6. Obesity.

Patients with diabetes have more extensive and more diffuse disease at an earlier age when compared with matched controls. More than 10% of the non-diabetic population over the age of 50 years have serious occult or overt atherosclerosis. More than 50% of the diabetic population are aged 65 years or over and it is not surprising that up to 60% have significant macrovascular disease two years after the diagnosis has been established.

9.2 REDUCING THE RISK

There is little we can do about ageing but smoking should be vigorously discouraged. Smoking outweighs all other risk factors for peripheral vascular disease in the diabetic. Smoking 10 cigarettes per day or more reduces the amputation age in men by 13 years and in women by 26 years! Smoking should not be allowed in health care areas and certainly not in hospitals. Governments could do much to help the situation and reduce the frightful mortality of the smoking related diseases by taxing smoking out of existence. The cost of smoking should be taken out of the cost of living index. It has nothing to do with living but more perhaps with the cost of dying. Unfortunately, governments have a vested interest.

Hypertension must be sought out and effectively treated. There is good evidence that control of hypertension reduces cerebrovascular episodes and may reduce the incidence of coronary thrombosis.

In the diabetic population it is essential to achieve normal or near normal glycaemia to reduce the risk factor.

In the past low-carbohydrate diets associated with a large fat intake probably raised serum lipid levels and predisposed to macrovascular disease. With modern high-fibre, high-carbohydrate, low-fat diets (see section 4.4) the serum cholesterol, triglycerides and obesity should be significantly reduced. If adherence to such a diet with weight reduction does not normalize serum lipids then lipid lowering agents should be given. Bezafibrate has the advantage of not only reducing the risk factor VLDL but also raises the protective factor HDL2. Cholestyramine and probucol are helpful in type 2 hyperlipidaemia. It must not be forgotten that patients with diabetes may also have a primary hyperlipidaemia.

Macrovascular disease has many manifestations according to the territory supplied by the affected vessel. The main subgroups are as follows:

1. Cerebrovascular disease:
   (i) Transient ischaemic attack.
   (ii) Completed stroke.
2. Coronary artery disease:
   (i) Angina.
   (ii) Myocardial infarction.
3. Peripheral vascular disease:
   (i) Intermittent claudication.
   (ii) Lower limb ischaemia.

9.3 CEREBROVASCULAR DISEASE

The screening process for cerebrovascular disease is as follows. It is based on a careful history and examination followed by appropriate investigation.

1. History:
   (i) Amaurosis fugax.

   (ii) Transient motor/sensory/speech disturbance.
   (iii) Transient vertigo.
   (iv) Completed stroke.
2. Examination:
   (i) Neurological signs.
   (ii) Cervical bruit.
   (iii) Blood pressure.
   (iv) Macrovascular disease at other sites.
3. Investigation:
   (i) Ultrasound.
   (ii) Digital subtraction angiography (IV, IA).
   (iii) Conventional angiography.
   (iv) CT brain scan.

Transient ischaemic episodes may present as amaurosis fugax, (transient recurrent loss of vision), transient motor, sensory or speech disturbance as the result of extracranial internal carotid artery disease. Transient vertigo may result from vertebrobasilar artery disease. Ischaemic episodes may pass unnoticed if emboli lodge in 'silent' areas of the brain or during sleep. CT brain scans often show multiple infarct areas in patients who have suffered only one transient ischaemic attack (TIA). In patients with ulcerated atheromatous plaques of the internal carotid artery, the incidence of multiple infarcts is 83% compared with only 19% in non-ulcerated plaques.

By definition, transient ischaemic attacks produce signs and symptoms for less than 24 hours. Signs of more than 24 hours duration indicate a completed stroke. However, only 50% of patients with a completed stroke have a warning TIA. The incidence of permanent neurological defect following a completed stroke is twice as great in the diabetic when compared with the non-diabetic.

Most strokes are caused by cerebral emboli originating from extracranial sites. Some are due to vascular thrombosis, others to cerebral haemorrhage. A history of transient ischaemic attacks, absent or poorly pulsating carotid arteries, or the presence of a cervical bruit should lead to further investigation. However, a bruit may not be present if the stenosis exceeds 85% and in 25% of patients with a bruit, no disease will be found. Nevertheless, the presence of a bruit is an important indication for further investigation since the stroke rate of bruit positive patients is 1–3% per annum compared with bruit negative patients of 0.3–1.5% per annum (Wolf *et al.*,

1981).

Modern non-invasive techniques for the investigation of carotid artery disease do not carry the risk (0.7% risk of stroke) of conventional arteriography. Conventional angiography has now been replaced by digital subtraction angiography (DSA – IV or IA) and by duplex scan and high resolution real time B mode ultrasound scanning. These imaging techniques not only provide 'road map' information but also indicate the degree of stenosis present and the presence or absence of plaque ulceration. The latter is important in relation to multiple infarcts (see above) and the greater the stenosis, the greater is the risk of a completed stroke or TIA.

Carotid endarterectomy is probably the treatment of choice for patients with TIAs due to ulcerated atheromatous plaques and after recovery from completed stroke due to carotid artery stenosis. The aim is to prevent subsequent stroke. Medical treatment is only partly effective. Aspirin and dipyridamole both reduce the incidence of transient ischaemic attacks but do not reduce the incidence of completed stroke. Anticoagulation reduces the incidence of both TIA and completed stroke by half for 2 years but after this the beneficial effects may be negated by an increase in the incidence of cerebral haemorrhage.

In untreated carotid artery disease presenting as TIAs the stroke risk is 7.5% per annum. The perioperative mortality of carotid endarterectomy is 1.2% and the early stroke rate is 4.8% i.e. 6% in the first year. Thereafter the stroke rate is 1.8% per annum, significantly better than in non-treated patients.

The treatment of asymptomatic patients with a carotid bruit is controversial and will not be discussed further (see further reading).

9.4 CORONARY ARTERY DISEASE

Coronary artery disease should be investigated and treated as in the non-diabetic. The presence of macrovascular disease in any other region is a good predictor of coronary artery disease. In patients with intermittent claudication, 80%, have significant coronary artery disease although less than 50% have a typical history. The detection of coronary artery disease in patients undergoing surgery for peripheral vascular disease is important since the perioperative mortality of 3–5% and the later (3 year) mortality of 30–40% associated with this type of surgery is mostly due to myocardial infarction.

Before peripheral vascular surgery, coronary artery assessment should therefore be undertaken. The screening process for coronary artery disease is as follows:

1. History:
   (i) Angina/atypical chest pain.
   (ii) Myocardial infarction.
   (iii) Macrovascular disease at other sites.
2. Examination – Macrovascular disease/blood pressure.
3. Resting ECG.
4. Stress ECG – selected patients.
5. Coronary angiography selected patients.

Patients with a history of angina, atypical chest pain, myocardial infarction or macrovascular disease at other sites should have a resting ECG. If the resting ECG is normal then a stress ECG should be performed in selected patients. The presence of electrocardiographic evidence of myocardial ischaemia at rest or on exercise is an indication for consideration of coronary angiography and coronary artery bypass surgery. The incidence of a positive stress ECG performed in asymptomatic patients with macrovascular disease elsewhere and with a normal resting ECG is 24%.

Perioperative mortality for coronary artery bypass surgery is now 2% and the 5-year mortality is 10%.

Myocardial infarction in the diabetic carries twice the mortality of the non-diabetic (28% vs. 14%) and warrants urgent admission to a coronary care unit. Metabolic control is often considerably upset during myocardial infarction. Control is best maintained using continuous low dose insulin infusion paying particular attention to serum potassium throughout. Disordered magnesium homeostasis is known to occur in myocardial infarction, particularly in diabetics. In non-diabetics, intravenous magnesium infusions during the first 48 hours post-infarct reduces the mortality and incidence of arrhythmias by more than half (Rasmussen *et al.*, 1986). An improvement in the prognosis for the diabetic may be achieved by similar means.

9.5 PERIPHERAL VASCULAR DISEASE

Peripheral vascular disease is manifest by the development of intermittent claudication and ischaemic changes in the legs and feet.

Because of its important and multifactorial causation, diabetic foot disease is considered in Chapter 11.

Screening for lower limb ischaemia may be summarized as follows:

1. History:
   (i) Intermittent claudication.
   (ii) Lower limb ulceration/slow healing.
   (iii) Rest pain.
   (iv) Macrovascular disease at other sites.
2. Examination:
   (i) Pulses.
   (ii) Dependent rubor.
   (iii) Ischaemic changes in skin and its appendages.
   (iv) Arterial bruit.
   (v) Ankle/arm Doppler pressure ratios (selected patients).
3. Investigations in selected patients:
   (i) Plain X-ray to show small vessel calcification.
   (ii) Tests for autonomic and peripheral neuropathy.
   (iii) Ultrasound.
   (iv) Digital subtraction angiography (IV, IA).
   (v) Conventional angiography.

A history of intermittent claudication, lower limb ulceration or slow healing indicates lower limb ischaemia. Intermittent claudication is characterized by pain, usually in the calf, coming on with exercise and relieved by rest. The claudicating distance is shortened by cold weather, and by ascending inclines and stairs. The claudicating distance is a useful measure of improvement or deterioration. Patients with intermittent claudication should be encouraged to take exercise since this may stimulate the growth of collateral vessels. The presence of rest pain is a poor prognostic sign. Macrovascular disease in other sites must be sought as lower limb ischaemia is rarely isolated.

Clinical examination may reveal diminished or absent pulses. The skin may be atrophic, cyanosed and poorly perfused, and exhibit dependent rubor. Nails may be dystrophic and there is often a loss of hair from the toes. Ulcers may be indolent and fail to heal. Arterial bruits may be heard over stenosed vessels. The Doppler ankle/arm pressure ratio is reduced and if less than 1.0, under-perfusion is indicated and the foot is at risk. Interpretation of the ankle/arm pressure ratios must be cautious in the presence of autonomic neuropathy and distal gangrene. Here AV shunting may give falsely high ratios. Autonomic neuropathy may be suspected if small artery calcification is present which may be demonstrated on plain X-rays. Arterialized blood found in dilated veins on the dorsum of the foot confirms the presence of AV shunting in autonomic neuropathy (Plate 19). Other signs of peripheral and autonomic neuropathy may be present (Chapter 10).

If available non-invasive ultrasound techniques should be used to determine the extent and distribution of the arterial lesions. Duplex scanning and high-resolution real-time B mode ultrasound provides information on morphology and function. Digital subtraction angiography (DSA IV or IA) may demonstrate popliteal, tibial and even pedal arteries which may not be visible with conventional angiography, particularly in the presence of gangrene or rest pain. This type of demonstration may lead to femoro-tibial bypass and limb salvage which would otherwise have not been done.

The determination of the extent and sites of arterial lesions is a prerequisite to treatment. Short arterial occulusion (less than 5 cm) and short stenotic lesions may initially be treated with percutaneous transluminal angioplasty (PTA). The aim is to defer or avoid complex expensive surgery. PTA now comprises 7% of all vascular intervention in the USA. This figure may rise to 40% in the future.

PTA has been used to dilate many vessels including the aorta, mesenteric artery, internal iliac arteries (for impotence), femoral arteries and fibromuscular disease or carotid arteries. Complications such as arterial thrombosis, embolism and haematoma occur in less than 10% and surgical intervention is required in 5% to rectify the complication. This is no worse than the complication rate seen in surgical reconstruction. It is of particular use as an initial treatment and in the high-risk patient.

Table 9.1 summarizes the 3-year patency of vessels following reconstruction surgery or PTA (Doubilet and Abrams, 1984). It represents the cumulative arterial patency in survivors. Although the success rate for PTA is only 75% of that of surgery, PTA is very cost effective. If PTA fails then the more expensive procedure of arterial reconstruction is available.

9.6 CONCLUSION: A PLAN OF ACTION

If we are to reduce the mortality and morbidity of macrovascular

Table 9.1 3-year patency following PTA or surgery

	Surgical (%)	*PTA (%)*
Aorto-iliac/aorto-femoral	90	
Iliac PTA		65
Femoro-popliteal	60	
Femoral PTA		42

Source: Doubilet and Abrams (1984).

disease in diabetics, a concerted effort and planned action is necessary. Treatable risk factors (section 9.1) should be looked for and vigorously treated. All patients require an annual check for the presence of macrovascular disease. Any patient presenting a suggestive history or examination (sections 9.3, 9.4 and 9.5) should be investigated as indicated. Early treatment should be the aim. PTA should be undertaken where applicable and if this fails, or is not applicable, early reconstructive surgery performed. By taking this course of action the serious consequences of macrovascular related disease might hopefully be avoided or at the very least delayed. We must develop what Myers and Nicolaides (1985) regard as the natural sequel to continued advances in the treatment of macrovascular disease:

> 'The first era of vascular surgery was dominated by the development of surgical techniques. The second era saw the emergence of non-invasive investigations. We are now entering a third era which concentrates on early detection of asymptomatic disease and better understanding of its natural history in relation to risk factors. We can now detect and grade not only symptomatic but also asymptomatic carotid, lower limb and coronary disease non invasively. This will not only benefit the individual patient because of a more cost effective and accurate diagnosis with minimal morbidity, but will also allow us to study the natural history and epidemiology of early atherosclerotic disease. **The natural sequel to this, the development of effective prevention that can be applied when the disease is in its asymptomatic stage, is no longer in the distant future.**'

REFERENCES AND FURTHER READING

Doubilet, P. and Abrams, H.L. (1984) The cost of under utilisation. Percutaneous transluminal angioplasty for peripheral vascular disease. *N. Eng. J. Med.*, **310**, 95–102.

Myers, K.A. and Nicolaides, A.N. (1985) New developments in arterial surgery. *Rec. Adv. Surg.*, **12**, 252–69.

Rasmussen, H.S., Norregård, P., Lindeneg, O., McNair, P., Backer, V. and Balslev, S. (1986) Intravenous magnesium infusion in acute myocardial infarction. *Lancet*, **i**, 234.

Wolf, P.A., Kannel, W.B., Sorley, P. and McNamara, P. (1981). Asymptomatic carotid bruit and risk of stroke. The Framingham Study. *J. Am. Med. Assoc.*, **245**, 1442–45.

· Ten ·

Diabetic neuropathy

10.1 INTRODUCTION

All tissues are affected by the metabolic disorders produced by the diabetic state. The metabolic changes are many and complex. Increased activity in the sorbitol pathway has been demonstrated with accumulation of sorbitol in both the lens (Chapter 7) and nervous tissue.

Diabetes affects all divisions of the nervous system. Although diabetic encephalopathy has been described there is some doubt about this as an entity and it is mainly the peripheral and autonomic nerves which are damaged by the deranged metabolic state. The pathological changes include segmental demyelination and axonal degeneration. The segmental demyelination combined with the loss of fast fibres in peripheral nerves is responsible for the electrophysiological changes of reduced conduction velocity. Changes sometimes observed in severe hyperglycaemia and ketoacidosis may be due to osmotic damage to the axon. In the long-term structural and biochemical changes are seen in nervous tissue. The myelin is abnormal in fatty acid composition and both sorbitol and fructose are found in excess.

Disordered metabolism is almost certainly responsible for the clinical picture of symmetrical polyneuropathy in a diabetic. However, vascular factors are thought to be responsible for isolated nerve lesions of sudden onset (mononeuritis and mononeuritis multiplex).

Diabetic neuropathy is common; 6% of diabetics in a large series had symptoms of neuropathy and 21% had signs (Pirart 1965, 1978). In the same series 10% of patients had evidence of neuropathy at diagnosis and this increased to 50% after 25 years duration.

10.2 CLINICAL MANIFESTATIONS OF DIABETIC NEUROPATHY

The clinical manifestations of diabetic neuropathy are as follows:

1. Symmetrical sensory polyneuropathy
2. Autonomic neuropathy:
   (i) Gastrointestinal tract – diabetic diarrhoea, gastroparesis/dilatation.
   (ii) Cardiovascular – postural hypotension, tachycardia, cardiorespiratory arrest.
   (iii) Sweating abnormality – Gustatory sweating.
   (iv) Genitourinary tract – Impotence, retrograde ejaculation, neurogenic bladder.
3. Mononeuritis and mononeuritis multiplex.
4. Diabetic amyotrophy.

Symmetrical sensory polyneuropathy is characterized by a loss of ankle jerks and a loss of vibration sense. When this becomes symptomatic the patient complains of numbness, paraesthesia and has symmetrical impairment of pain and light touch sensation. In rare cases the loss of pain sensation may be associated with the development of a neuropathic arthropathy (Charcot joint). Neuropathic arthropathy in the diabetic commonly affects the foot, ankle and occasionally the knee. This is different to that seen in tabes dorsalis where the knee, hip and spine are most commonly affected. A loss of pain sensation is also often accompanied by painless perforating ulcers. This subject will be dealt with in Chapter 11.

Autonomic neuropathy has many different manifestations.

Diarrhoea (particularly nocturnal) is the commonest manifestation of autonomic neuropathy affecting the gastrointestinal tract. Gastroparesis may be associated with gross gastric dilatation, vomiting, and intractable hiccoughs.

Of the cardiovascular manifestations, postural hypotension and rhythm abnormalities are common. Postural hypotension may be defined as a fall in the systolic blood pressure of greater than 30 mm Hg on standing. This is why it is important to measure the blood pressure of the patient in both the lying and standing positions. High resting pulse rate is also common as is a fixed heart rate with no beat to beat variation. Cardiorespiratory arrest has been described and unexplained sudden death, particularly after surgery has been cited as a manifestation of autonomic neuropathy.

Sweating abnormalities and in particular gustatory sweating are often very distressing. In this manifestation of autonomic neuropathy profuse sweating occurs when food is either tasted or even only when an aroma is appreciated.

Impotence is common in diabetics. However, it must not be assumed that it is necessarily due to autonomic neuropathy. In many cases the restoration of physical fitness, plenty of reassurance, and if necessary psychosexual counselling will restore the patient's ability to perform.

Retrograde ejaculation may be caused by autonomic neuropathy. It must be considered as a possibility when investigating the infertile couple when the husband is a diabetic with other manifestations of neuropathy. Neurogenic bladder may contribute to genitourinary tract infection and chronic renal failure.

Mononeuropathy and multineuropathy (mononeuritis multiplex) are common in the elderly. Particularly common are the cranial neuropathies affecting the third and fourth ocular motor nerves. Such neuropathies are acute in onset and are sometimes associated with pain. There is a gradual recovery over the course of weeks or at the most months. Interestingly, in third nerve mononeuropathy the pupillomotor function is spared. Peripheral nerves, particularly the femoral nerve and the lateral popliteal nerve are also affected. The latter produces foot drop.

Diabetic amyotrophy first described by Garland and Tavener (Garland and Tavener, 1953) is a neuropathy affecting diabetic patients in middle or later life. The diabetes is usually of short duration. There is asymmetric proximal muscle wasting and weakness. The muscles of the pelvic girdle and thighs are most commonly affected although the shoulders and the arms may be similarly affected. The neuropathy is accompanied by pain. The reflexes are diminished and the plantar responses may be extensor. The CSF contains an increased concentration of protein. There is usually a slow and spontaneous recovery with good diabetic control.

10.3 SCREENING FOR DIABETIC NEUROPATHY

The screening programme for diabetic neuropathy is set out below:

1. History:
   (i) Sensory symptoms – pain/paraesthesia/numbness.
   (ii) Motor symptoms – foot drop/diplopia.
   (iii) Symptoms of autonomic neuropathy
2. Examination:
   (i) Loss of ankle reflexes.
   (ii) Diminution/loss – light touch, pain, vibration sense.
   (iii) Signs of autonomic neuropathy.
3. Investigations:
   (i) Vibration threshold (Biosthesiometer, Bloom *et al.*, 1984)
   (ii) Electrophysiology : nerve conduction studies (selected patients).

Screening for diabetic autonomic neuropathy.

1. History:
   (i) Sweating abnormalities.
   (ii) Impotence.
   (ii) Retrograde ejaculation.
   (iv) Vomiting and diarrhoea (particularly nocturnal).
2. Examination:
   (i) Pupillary abnormalities (small/irregular/unequal or unreactive to light).
   (ii) Tachycardia/bradycardia.
   (iii) Postural hypotension.
   (iv) Sweating abnormalities, e.g. gustatory sweating, dry foot with fissuring.
3. Investigations:
   (i) Beat-to-beat variation.
   (ii) Dorsal foot vein blood gases to detect arterialized venous blood.
   (iii) Plain X-rays to detect small vessel calcification.

It is based on a careful history and clinical examination followed by selective investigation.

The detection of autonomic neuropathy should warn anaesthetists of the potential danger of cardiorespiratory arrest. The detection of diabetic neuropathy in general has important implications in relation to diabetic foot disease (see Chapter 11).

At early stage diabetic neuropathy is reversible. Good glycaemic control may well reverse and will almost certainly delay the progress of diabetic neuropathy.

Early detection of diabetic neuropathy will be an added stimulus to both patient and the health care team to achieve normal or near normal glycaemia.

10.4 TREATMENT

The treatment of diabetic neuropathy is problematic. No definite and specific treatments have yet been described. Good glycaemic control seems to be the best way of avoiding diabetic neuropathy and treating it should it occur. Other factors contributing to a neuropathy such as B_{12} deficiency or excess alcohol should be corrected. Painful symptomatic neuropathy has been treated with diphenylhydantoin (Epanutin), multivitamin injection, carbamazepine (Tegretol), and low dose aspirin. None of the above symptomatic treatments are of proven use.

Postural hypotension has been treated with fludrocortisone 0.4 mg daily. Unfortunately all treatments for postural hypotension appear to be singularly ineffective and complicated by side effects.

Gustatory sweating may sometimes be helped by anticholinergic agents such as poldine methylsulphate, 2–4 mg three times daily.

Some patients with autonomic neuropathy develop resistant oedema which is occasionally helped by ephedrine hydrochloride 30–60 mg three times daily. Side effects are common.

The treatment of diabetic gastroparesis with oral domperidone looks promising (Watts *et al*,, 1985). It also appears to have some effect on diabetic diarrhoea. Domperidone is taken in a dose of 10 mg four times a day by mouth.

The treatment of diabetic neuropathy is unsatisfactory. Prevention is undoubtedly better than cure and monitoring the standard of control and maintaining good glycaemic control is the best form of insurance.

REFERENCES AND FURTHER READING

Bloom, S., Till, S., Sonksen, P. and Smith, S. (1984) Use of a biosthesiometer to measure individual vibration thresholds and their variation in 519 non diabetic subjects. *Bri. Med. J.*, **288**, 1793–5.

Garland, H. and Taverner, D. (1953) Diabetic myelopathy. *Br. Med. J.*, **i**, 1405–8.

Keen, H. and Jarrett, R.J. (eds) (1982) *Complications of Diabetes*, 2nd edn. Edward Arnold, London.

Pirart, J. (1965) Diabetic neuropathy: a metabolic or a vascular disease? *Diabetes*, **14**, 1.

Pirart, J. (1978) *Diabetes Care*, **1**, 168–252.

Watts, G.F., Armitage, M., Sinclair, J. and Hill, R.D. (1985) Treatment of diabetic gastroparesis with oral domperidone. *Diab. Med.*, **ii**, 491.

· Eleven ·

Diabetic foot disease

11.1 INTRODUCTION

In diabetic foot disease the various pathological processes conspire together to inflict damage to the patient's tissues which may eventually result in the necessity for amputation. The various components of this process are as follows:

1. Macrovascular disease:
   (i) Localized.
   (ii) Diffuse.
2. Microvascular disease.
3. Autonomic neuropathy.
4. Peripheral neuropathy.
5. Infection.

Macrovascular disease decreases the blood supply to the foot. Microvascular disease reduces tissue perfusion at the capillary level. Autonomic neuropathy produces AV shunting, again diverting blood away from tissues. The loss of pain sensation (sensory polyneuropathy) deprives the patient of the normal protection from noxious stimuli. Minor trauma and infection go unheeded and painless neuropathic perforating ulcers result. Hyperglycaemia decreases the host's ability to resist infection by both fungi and bacteria. Infections spread rapidly through the debilitated tissues.

The end-result of these pathological processes produces an incidence of gangrene which is at least 20 times greater in the diabetic when compared with the non-diabetic. In the USA, 11.5% of all diabetic admissions are due to foot problems; and of all American diabetics, 5–15% will require amputation. Sadly within 5 years, 51% well require a second amputation. In this group between 41 and 70% of patients survive less than 5 years. Of all admissions to the Joselin Clinic for Diabetes, 25% are for diabetic foot disease. No less than 40% require amputation with a 5% mortality despite optimal medical and surgical care.

Neuropathic and ischaemic processes may affect the foot to varying degrees. Patients may develop a predominantly neuropathic or ischaemic foot. However, many patients have a combination of both.

11.2 THE NEUROPATHIC FOOT

The manifestations of neuropathic foot disease are caused by unperceived noxious mechanical, chemical, or thermal stimuli. In the non-neuropathic situation, even minimal discomfort is rapidly counteracted by adjustment of position. In the absence of pain sensation trauma continues and no adjustment is made. This is particularly so when the trauma is mechanical. The commonest mechanical trauma affecting the foot is pressure. This may be vertical as the weight of the body is transferred via the foot to the ground, or sheer due to rubbing of ill fitting footwear (Plate 20). Sheer forces are maximum with jogging, running or walking with long strides, and minimum with walking and short strides.

Pressure = force/area, therefore, if the weight of the body is distributed over a large area of the foot the pressure is low. However, in the presence of neuropathy and/or deformity (see below) the weight may be transmitted through a localized area producing high pressure.

The following foot deformities predispose patients to diabetic foot disease:

1. Pes cavus (high arched foot).
2. Flat feet.
3. Claw toes.
4. Hammer toes.
5. Mallet toes.
6. Hallux valgus (bunion) (Plate 20).
7. Tailor's bunion (bunionette).
8. Hallux rigidus.

High pressure areas may be demonstrated by using a pedobarograph or Harris's mat. These simple instruments demonstrate areas of high pressure generated in the foot on standing and walking.

High- pressure areas stimulate callous formation. An ulcer is usually preceded by haematoma or area of fat necrosis as a result of trauma or pressure. The centre of the overlying skin becomes ischaemic, and this results in an ulcer with undermined and calloused edges. This punched-out lesion is usually found on the plantar surface of the foot. It is most commonly seen under the head of the first or other metatarasals. However, other common sites are on the heel and on the dorsum and tips of the toes. The ulcer is usually surrounded by a thick layer of callous and does not heal. It is painless and penetrates deep into tissues and may even affect bone.

Although the ulceration is painless the patient may complain of neuropathic foot pain. This has a particularly burning or lancenating quality which is often worse at night. Parasthesiae and hypersensitivity are not uncommon and even the bed clothes touching the skin of the neuropathic foot will keep the patient awake.

Neuropathy may also cause weakness of the intrinsic muscles of the foot and produce clawing of the toes.

Autonomic neuropathy affecting the foot produces inappropriate under- or over-capillary perfusion. Arteriovenous shunts also divert blood from the capillary bed to the post-capillary veins. This causes a rise in post-capillary venous pressure which in turn raises the capillary pressure. Increased capillary pressure increases the rate of transudation and interstitial oedema results. The resulting poor capillary flow produces stasis and an increased risk of infection and ulceration. The presence of autonomic neuropathy may give rise to a bounding peripheral pulse. This may lull the physician into a false sense of security and lead him to assume that tissue perfusion is adequate. AV shunting may be inferred from the presence of a bounding peripheral pulse, dilated veins on the dorsum of the foot, and the presence of arterialized blood in these veins (Plate 19).

Rarely the foot may be disorganized further by the development of neuropathic (Charcot) joints (Plate 21).

11.3 THE ISCHAEMIC FOOT

The ischaemic foot is characterized by pain. Exercise may produce intermittent claudication and certainly makes the foot pain worse. A significant deterioration in the condition is heralded by pain occurring at rest. Often the pain keeps the patient awake at night and is relieved to some extent by hanging the leg over the side of the bed. Ischaemic ulceration is typically painful and shows poor granulation. There is little healing and the dead gangrenous edge to the ulcer is seen in contrast to the prolific callous formation of the neuropathic ulcer. The toes of the severely ischaemic foot tend to shrink, blacken and may undergo autoamputation (Plate 22).

11.4 ASSESSMENT OF THE DIABETIC FOOT

This is summarized below:

1. Clinical history and examination:
   (i) Symptoms and signs of ischaemia (see section 9.5).
   (ii) Symptoms and signs of neuropathy (see section 10.3).
   (iii) Infection
   (iv) Ulceration.
2. Simple in-clinic foot laboratory investigation:
   (i) Ankle/arm Doppler pressure ratio.
   (ii) Vibration sense (biosthesiometer).
   (iii) Pedobarograph.
3. Other investigations:
   (i) Plain X-rays
   (ii) Ultrasound
   (iii) Angiography
   (iv) The future – transcutaneous oximetry and laser Doppler capillary flowmetry.
4. Footwear assessment.

Symptoms suggesting ischaemia and neuropathy should be sought. Palpation of the pulses will give an indication of the state of the major vessels. The presence or absence of ankle reflex, light touch, pain sensation and vibration sense will indicate the presence or absence of neuropathy. Evidence of bacterial and fungal infection, particularly in the interdigital clefts should be sought.

If significant disease is found then further investigation is indicated.

At the bedside an ankle/arm systolic blood pressure ratio may be measured. Similarly the vibration sense may be objectively assessed using a biosthesiometer (Bloom *et al.*, 1984). Areas of high pressure may be inferred from the presence of callous or detailed using the pedobarograph or Harris's mat.

X-rays of the legs and feet will indicate the presence of calcification in major and small vessels of the foot. It will also indicate the presence of infection in bone. An isotopic bone scan may be of value.

Ultrasound Doppler imaging is a useful non-invasive technique for the assessment of large blood vessels. It should be used to define those patients with localized blocks which are possibly amenable to surgery. Those patients with localized blocks should undergo angiography with a view to surgical intervention (Chapter 9). In the future transcutaneous oximetry and laser Doppler flowmetry may be a useful adjunct in the assessment of patients with diabetic foot disease.

The standard of biochemical control should be assessed in terms of home blood glucose monitoring, laboratory interval blood sugar, and HbA1. The serum lipids should be measured although intervention at this stage is unlikely to affect the outcome. The haematocrit (packed cell volume PCV) should be assessed since a PCV greater than 45% significantly reduces blood flow due to increased whole blood viscosity.

If infection is present an attempt should be made to isolate the organism. Callouses should be removed and swabs taken.

Common anaerobic organisms are found in deep infections. Bacteriodes and *Clostridium perfringens* are common. The latter may produce gas. Similarly *E. coli*, streptococci and staphylococci are also found. The danger of a life-threatening septicaemia is ever present in the debilitated patient with a septic foot.

The importance of apparently innocuous fungal infections of the foot must not be overlooked. Tinea pedis (interdigital) due to trichophyton and *Candida albicans* may produce enough damage to the skin to provide a portal of entry for more serious organisms.

11.5 MANAGEMENT

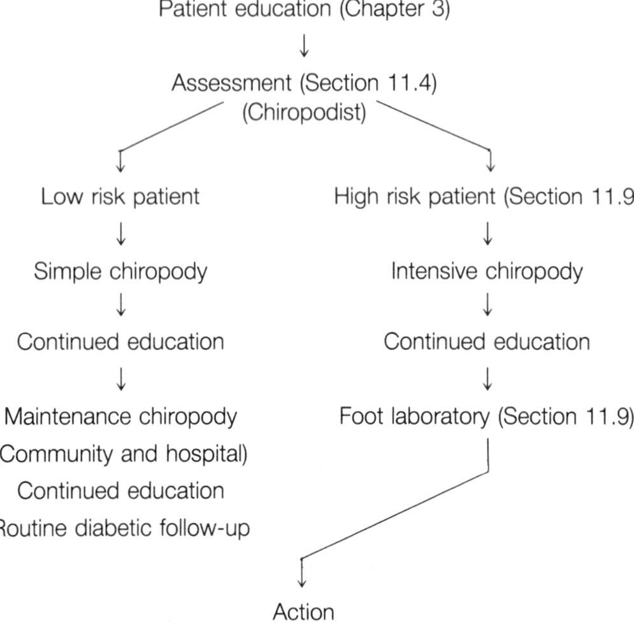

To treat foot deformity (orthopaedic surgeon/chiropodist)
To treat ischaemia (radiologist/vascular surgeon)
To treat neuropathy (physician)
To treat ulceration/infection (chiropodist, surgeon, nurse, physician)
Maintenance chiropody
Protective footwear (chiropodist, orthotist, shoemaker)
Maintenance of normal or near normal glycaemia

Figure 11.1 The prevention and management of diabetic foot disease.

11.5.1 The prevention of diabetic foot ulceration

Prevention of diabetic foot ulceration may be summarized as follows:

1. Patient education : foot care
2. Good glycaemic control.
3. Normolipidaemia.

4. Avoidance of smoking.
5. Exercise.
6. Footwear.
7. Chiropody.

If amputation is to be avoided, the presence of neuropathic and/or ischaemic features must be taken very seriously (Plate 23). The patient must be taught how to look after the vulnerable foot and intensive follow up undertaken. The aim is to conserve and management should be conservative.

Foot care education should be introduced shortly after the diagnosis of diabetes and be reinforced throughout. A set of instructions should be given to the patient (see also *Have Healthy Feet* by Lyn Cheater (1986), useful reading for patients and health care workers):

1. Wash the feet every day and dry carefully between the toes. Inspect your feet daily using a miror if necessary or ask someone else to check them for you. The feet should not be 'soaked'. A light dusting of non-medicated talc may be used. A simple aqueous cream (e.g. E.45 – Crookes Products) may be applied to the skin – but not between the toes.
2. Cut toe-nails straight across, after washing the feet. If your sight is not good, do not attempt to use scissors on your feet, but go to the chiropodist regularly. Tell him you are diabetic.
3. Do not walk about bare-footed, especially on wooden floors.
4. Corn paint, plasters, salves or pads should not be used.
5. Make sure that your shoes fit and have broad toes and low heels and do not wear new shoes for more than half-an-hour at a time. Stockings and socks should be of natural fibre (cotton or wool).
6. Avoid excessive heat and cold. To avoid cold, wear thick socks, preferably clean every day and long pants. Never put your feet close, or nearer than 4 ft (1¼ m) to the fire. Remove hot water bottles from the bed before getting in.
7. Report all sore places, blisters, or discoloured areas to the doctor, however trivial they may seem to you.
8. Do not smoke.
9. By obeying these simple rules, the majority of serious foot troubles will be avoided.

Revision should take place when there is any suspicion of diabetic foot disease developing. Particular attention should be given to footwear. No smoking must be strongly advised. Good glycaemic control is essential and adherence to a high-fibre low-fat diet advised. An attempt should be made to maintain serum lipids within the normal range from diagnosis.

Regular chiropody must be provided and the patient should be taught to wash and inspect the feet daily. Certain patients may find a mirror useful in inspecting the feet. If vision is poor or difficulty is experienced somebody else should check the feet daily. Particular attention should be paid to the interdigital clefts and fungal infections treated early. Trichophyton infections should be treated with Whitfield's Ointment or clotrimazole. Candida infections should be treated with miconazole. Regular examination by a nurse or doctor must be arranged. An alternative to beta blockade should be used in the treatment of hypertension.

If there is clinical evidence of macrovascular disease, early investigation and intervention should be the rule. In the presence of localized blocks transluminal angioplasty should be tried and if not effective then reconstructive surgery considered.

11.5.2 The management of established diabetic foot disease in the presence of ulceration and infection

All callouses and dead skin must be removed and extensive debridement undertaken. Swabs should be taken and sent to microbiology. Adequate drainage is essential. All undermined skin must be removed and the ulcer completely saucerized so that epithelialization can occur from the edges.

For minor changes the patient may be allowed home to rest the leg. All patients with plantar ulcers need to be off weight bearing until the ulcer has healed. A less certain way to remove the pressure from such a lesion in order to promote healing is by the contact skin plaster. Daily dressings using Eusol (0.25% hypochlorite) and paraffin or glycerine and magnesium sulphate should be tried. Oral antibiotics may be given at this stage.

11.5.3 Indications for admission

The presence of acute infection, the necessity for surgical intervention, poor diabetic (glycaemic) control are absolute indications for admission. Poor domestic circumstances and the lack of services within the community are relative indications for admission. Bed rest is essential.

Following extensive debridement and open drainage, antibiotics such as benzyl penicillin 1 mega unit six hourly and flucloxacillin 500 mg six hourly should be given intravenously. Metronidazole 200 mg orally six hourly or 1 g per rectum should be given eight hourly. Wounds should be cleaned by irrigating with sodium hypochlorite (1% w/v stabilized in sodium chloride). If these measures fail to control the infection then amputation may become necessary as a life saving measure. Meddlesome nibbling and multiple conservative amputation should be avoided. A definitive operation should be carried out at the appropriate level.

Amputation as an end-result of diabetic foot disease represents a failure in medical treatment. Many amputations could be avoided by patient education, a good chiropody service, and a good shoe fitting service. A failure to appreciate these simple facts results in amputation with its attendant cost and suffering. Resources used for patient education, chiropody services, and shoe fitting services prove very cost effective.

11.6 CHIROPODY SERVICE

In the UK, the chiropodists/podiatrist must receive a basic training which would enable registration under The Professions Supplementary to Medicine Act (1966). In other countries or states equivalent training and registration should be obtained.

The chiropodist should not be purely interventionist, treating the patients when trouble arises. The various parts played by the chiropodist in an organised health care system are as follows:

1. Patient education.
2. Initial assessment.
3. Intensive treatment.
4. Foot laboratory.
5. Footwear assessment and fitting.
6. Follow-up maintenance (as necessary).
7. Domiciliary service.

The patient's initial contact with the chiropodist should be during a diabetic education session (see Chapter 3). This should be followed by an assessment session (see sections 11.4 and *Figure 11.1*). During this session, education on a one-to-one basis should continue and careful assessment of the suitability of the patient's footwear and personal foot care made. The aim should be to detect the high-risk patient (see section 11.9). Routine follow-up maintenance and review should be organized as necessary. For the elderly and infirm, a domiciliary service is essential.

The staffing of the chiropody service is an important but neglected aspect of diabetic care. There are no national norms for chiropody staffing in the United Kingdom. In 1978 The Society of Chiropodists in the UK suggested a staffing norm of one chiropodist and one foot care assistant per 2000 elderly population. Remembering that more than 50% of the diabetic population are over the age of 65 years, this would suggest that at least one whole-time chiropodist together with one whole-time foot care assistant would be required to service a diabetic population of 2500 derived from a general population of 250 000. These sessions might be deployed as follows:

1. Staffing levels: one chiropodist and one foot care assistant per 2000 diabetics.
2. Chiropodist: sessions (10 session week); each week :
   1 Education session (See chapter 3).
   2 Assessment session (e.g. new patients and foot laboratory).
   2 Intensive treatment sessions (often with joint consultation with diabetic clinic staff).
   3 Maintenance follow-up sessions (routine chiropody).
   1 Domiciliary session (home visits for the elderly).
   1 Administration and teaching session.
3. Foot care assistant: Sessions : 10 session week under the supervision and direction of the chiropodist. The distribution of sessions must be flexible to suit local needs and conditions.

The chiropodist must work in close association with the shoe-fitting service.

11.7 DIABETIC SHOE-FITTING SERVICE

The provision of therapeutic and protective footwear is an important part of any diabetic service. Despite this, most diabetologists have little knowledge of the subject. There is tremendous scope for co-operation between physician, chiropodist, orthotist (the person who actually measures the feet and provides the shoe maker with vital information) and the shoemaker, and yet joint consultation rarely if ever takes place. It is the physician and chiropodist working together who will be able to define clearly the exact characteristics of the footwear required. These characteristics must then be discussed with the orthotist who will make the vital measurements for the shoemaker to act upon. Finally the manufacturer must be made to realize that the footwear required is that which was defined by the physician and chiropodist and not a preconceived 'orthopaedic shoe'.

Tovey (Tovey, 1985) has established a diabetic shoe service second to none in the UK. He has called upon his extensive experience in treating patients with neuropathic foot disease due to leprosy in India in 1951–1968 and has formulated the minimum requirements for a diabetic shoe as follows:

1. The shoes must be deep enough to accomodate the thickness of the required cushioning insole. They should be lace-up, with low heels and wide waists. The toes must be broad and the toe spaces large enough to avoid pressure on clawed toes. The uppers (and their lining) must be made of the thinnest leather available. Toe puffs (stiffening) must be omitted and heel stiffening reduced.
2. When there is sensory loss without any high-pressure areas a soft Poron open cell rubber cushioning insole is required. For an average weight patient a 9 mm thickness insole is necessary. Heavier patients require a 13 mm insole and for a lighter patient a 6 mm insole will be sufficient.
3. If there are localized pressure points cradles are required to redistribute the weight bearing. Pressure areas may be inferred from the appearance of the foot and from callous formation. They may be defined more accurately using a pedobarograph or Harris's mat. In the past cradles were made of cork but now high-density Plastazote is used. After heating in a hot air oven this is moulded to the last under pressure which reduces the thickness from 13 to 6 mm. Cut-outs or sinks are made under the pressure areas defined as above and these are filled with 6 mm Neoprene cushioning. The whole cradle is then covered with an 8 mm cushioning of Neoprene. Neoprene is chosen

because it is a closed-cell microcellular rubber and does not 'bottom out' under high pressure. It is firmer than Poron.

Special shoes are designed to prevent ulcers occurring or recurring after healing. All ulcers must be healed beforehand. They will not heal if the patient is weight bearing. Exceptionally weight bearing may be allowed with a total contact plaster.

11.8 COSTS

To obtain funds for preventative medicine it is necessary to show that it is cost effective. In this context it is worthwhile reiterating statistics quoted earlier in this chapter. Of all diabetic admissions in the USA, 11.5% are due to foot problems. Of all diabetics in the USA, 5–15% will require amputation. The provision of an open access service with 24 hour telephone cover staffed by specialist nurses and associated with an improved chiropody service has been shown to be very cost effective. The amputation rate may be reduced by as much as 50% and the length of stay in hospital by 85% (Davidson, 1983; Miller *et al.*, 1981).

The annual cost of diabetic foot disease in the USA is estimated to be in excess of 100 million dollars. A study in Nottingham (UK) suggested the need for 7000 more chiropodists and indicated that there was a potential saving of 15 million pounds. Even a small saving would pay the salaries of the many chiropodists and specialist nurses needed.

11.9 A PLAN OF ACTION

The setting up of a comprehensive service for the prevention and treatment of diabetic foot disease requires a plan of action. Such a plan is outlined as follows:

1. Formulate a definite and clear foot care policy.
2. Education:
   (i) Staff.
   (ii) Patient.
3. Assessment : detection of high-risk patient.
4. Establish a routine chiropody service with open referral (in hospital and community).
5. Establish an intensive chiropody service and diabetic foot laboratory.

6. Define links with radiologist, physicist, vascular surgeon, orthopaedic surgeon, chiropodist, orthotist, shoemaker.
7. Establish a footwear service.

The first essential is to formulate a definite and clear foot care policy for the district and ensure that all staff are aware of and adhere to the policy.

Education, like charity, should begin at home. The diabetologist must be well versed in what is involved. He must then set out a comprehensive programme of education for nursing, chiropody and medical staff. It should not be forgotten that the service extends out into the community and is not confined to the hospital. The education programme must therefore extend to family doctors and other workers in the community.

Education of the patient is paramount. Advice on foot care should start early in the educational programme and should be continued during chiropody assessment and follow-up.

An early assessment should be made to detect the high-risk patient. A combination of initial medical review and chiropody assessment should detect the patient at risk. The factors characterizing the high-risk patient are as follows:

1. Neuropathy.
2. Ischaemia – smoking (past or present).
3. Deformity.
4. Infection (fungal/bacterial).
5. Poor hygiene.
6. Poor grasp of foot care education.
7. Poor glycaemic control.
8. Obesity.
9. Increasing age.
10. Low social status (group).

It is important to establish an effective routine chiropody service both in the hospital and in the community.

High-risk patients and patients with established diabetic foot disease require more intensive chiropody and more detailed assessment. This requirement is probably best satisfied by the development of a diabetic foot laboratory staffed by especially trained chiropodists. The function of the diabetic foot laboratory is as follows:

1. Intensive chiropody/clinical assessment.
2. Ankle/arm pressure ratio (Doppler).
3. Vibration threshold (biosthesiometer).
4. Pressure area assessment (pedobarograph).
5. Joint consultation (chiropodist/orthotist/physician.
6. Preparation and fitting protective footwear and appliances.

11.10 CONCLUSION

The task of setting up an effective service to deal with diabetic foot disease is enormous. However, the task cannot be avoided since the neglect of this important aspect of diabetic care will bring untold suffering to patients and high costs to the health service.

REFERENCES AND FURTHER READING

Bloom, S., Till, S., Sonksen, P. and Smith, S. (1984) Use of a biothesiometer to measure individual vibration thresholds and their variation in 519 non-diabetic subjects. *Br. Med. J.*, **288**, 1793.

Davidson, J.K. (1983) *The Grady Memorial Hospital Diabetes Unit Ambulatory Care Programme*. Excerpta Medica International Congress Series No. 624, pp. 286–97.

Miller, L.V., Goldstein, J., Kumar, D. and Dye, L. (1981) Assessment of programme effectiveness at the Los Angeles County – University of Southern California Medical Centre. In *Educating Diabetic Patients* (eds G. Steiner and P.A. Lawrence) Springer, New York, pp. 349–59.

Tovey, F.I. (1984) The manufacture of diabetic footwear. *Diab. Med.*, **1**, 69–71.

Tovey, F.I. (1985) Establishing a diabetic shoe service. *Practical Diabetes*, **2**, 3–5.

Tovey, F.I. (1986) Care of the diabetic foot. *Practical Diabetes*, **3**, 130–34.

Good reading for health care workers and patients alike: *Have Healthy Feet* Lyn Cheater (Javlin Book, 1986).

· Twelve ·

The role of the nurse in diabetes

R.D. Hill in association with P. Diment SRN (Diabetic Ward Sister) and P. Hindley SRN (Diabetic Liaison Sister)

12.1 INTRODUCTION

Nursing had its origins in antiquity with the development of hospitals and hospices as a refuge for the weak and hospitality for the stranger. The coming of Christianity to Rome with its Roman converts brought a strong religious element into nursing which carried on into the monastic organizations of the dark ages. It was from the monastic orders that primitive health services radiated.

It was the development of military and chivalric orders that originated the charitable hospitals. The Knights of St. John built two hospitals in Jerusalem and branches spread throughout the world. It was here that the hierarchical organization of nursing care had its roots. However, at this time volunteerism began with its sense of a calling or vocation.

There was little further development until the beginning of the scientific explosion of medical knowledge in the sixteenth century. William Harvey was at the forefront of this activity which was given new impetus with the development of the germ theory in the nineteenth century.

Florence Nightingale appeared on the scene in the UK in the nineteenth century. In 1854 she went to the Crimea to sort out what can only be described as a medical disaster. Her success can be judged on basic statistics. She reduced the death rate amongst the sick and wounded from 50 to 2.5%. Public imagination was fired and public subscription funded the School of Nursing at St. Thomas's Hospital in London. A revolution in nursing care in England had begun, and within 25 years the face of nursing in England was totally changed.

In 1919 the Nursing Act was passed and the General Nursing Council formed with provision for the Registration for Nurses.

In 1946 a comprehensive system of health care was developed in the UK known as the National Health Service.

World-wide demand for improved medical care has increased rapidly during the last 40 years. Expectations in relation to what can be achieved medically have increased. At the same time there has been an increase in materialism with a readiness to take legal action against perceived malpractice. This has been a particular problem in the USA. Increasing health care demands and expectations have been associated with important changes in the role of the nurse.

12.2 SPECIALIZATION

In the United Kingdom basic educational requirements are needed before entry into a School of Nursing. In the School of Nursing a general training is pursued covering all aspects of theoretical and practical nursing. Students graduate by obtaining a general nursing qualification (in the UK, enrolled nurse or a Registered General Nurse in 1986). After qualification many nurses continue in general nursing. Others continue to study for higher qualifications and specialize as midwives or community nurses. The fields of specialization are many and varied. Some fields require detailed expert knowledge in a limited field such as coronary care and intensive care. Others requires special expertise in general nursing for special groups e.g. in paediatrics. In all specialized areas there are courses, in-service training, and in some cases higher qualifications. Nurses are expected to acquire managerial skills and run a ward or a group of wards.

During the last 40 years, technical advances have accelerated the process of specialization and resulted in an extended role for the nurse. In addition to the usually well-recognized specialities a new branch of the nursing profession has become more clearly defined.

In 1940, because of severe wartime bed shortage in Leicestershire, Dr Bailey organized the first community based specialist nursing service for diabetics in the United Kingdom (if not for the world). The organization has been continued and developed by Dr John Hernshaw. In this service specialized, highly qualified nurses (health visitors) take on the role of advisers to diabetics in the community. Both children and adults are managed at home from the outset whether or not they require insulin. The nurses are experts in the field of diabetes and with the physician provide an excellent 24-hour service.

At the Grady Memorial Hospital in the United States nurse specialization was carried even further in the Ambulatory Care Programme. In this programme the patient's primary contact was with the nurse and each nurse had about 500 patients under her care (Davidson, 1983).

In the Karolinski Hospital in Sweden diabetes nurse specialists have developed the specialty further and provide a 5 day school for diabetics.

The development of the role of clinical nurse specialist with a special interest in one subject was officially recognized in the United Kingdom by the Royal College of Nursing in 1971. Several specialities have now been recognized:

1. Diabetic.
2. Paediatric.
3. Oncology.
4. Stoma.
5. Breast service.
6. Parenteral nutrition.
7. Continence.
8. Control of infection.

There has been some resistance to this development, not only from some physicians who felt threatened, but also from nurses who felt similarly threatened by a new race of 'specialists'.

12.3 THE ROLE OF THE NURSE IN DIABETES

The nurse occupies a central and key role in all aspects of diabetic care.

Those groups of nurses requiring training in diabetes are as follows:

1. District or community nurse.
2. Practice linked nurses.
3. Diabetic clinic (outpatient department) nurse or day hospital nurse.
4. Ward staff.
5. Clinical nurse specialist in diabetics:
   (i) Diabetic ward sister.
   (ii) Diabetic liaison sister.

12.3.1 The district or community nurse

The role of the district or community nurse in diabetic care is crucial. She will often be the first health care worker to detect a new diabetic by suspecting the diagnosis in an elderly patient, perhaps with an ulcerated leg. She will have frequent, often daily, contact with patients. She will be required to treat wounds and ulcers, monitor blood glucose, give insulin injections, and generally continue patients' education and give advice. She is not in general asked to adjust insulin doses. Because of the nature of her work she may feel isolated from other members of the diabetic health care team. If the health care team is to speak with one voice the organization must facilitate contact with other health care team members and provide suitable update education sessions. The clinical nurse specialist acting as a diabetic liaison sister can play an important part here.

12.3.2 The practice linked nurse

The practice linked nurse is employed by the family doctor and the work schedule is organized in conjunction with the family doctor concerned. This is a vital role in the routine follow-up of diabetics not attending the diabetic clinic (see chapters 6 and 13).

The clinical expertise and organizational ability will make or break the family doctor's efforts to organize diabetic care in general practice. The nurse must have special knowledge and training and form contacts with other members of the health care team.

Section 6.3 outlines what might be expected of the practice linked nurse. To this might be added the importance of organizing and managing a follow-up appointments system and the continued education of the diabetic. Once again if the whole service is to speak with one voice it is essential that the practice linked nurse is fully aware of what is taught in the diabetic education session and what the views of the health care team are. During the nurse follow-up interview the patient and relatives will talk to the nurse and will often confide and question the nurse rather than 'bother the doctor'. Consistent advice must be given by the whole health care team to avoid confusion.

12.3.3 The diabetic clinic, diabetic day hospital, and general ward nurses

The role of the nurse in the diabetic clinic is similar to that of the practice linked nurse. She should not be used as a mere usher to bring patients from the waiting room to see the doctor and usher them out again. She is expected to organize the collection of urine specimens (e.g. MSU) and the testing of urine. She should be responsible for weighing the patient and for measuring the blood pressure in the lying and standing position. She should be capable of measuring distant visual acuity and dilating the pupils as and when necessary. She should be able to examine the feet and bring any problems to the attention of the doctor. She should have sufficient knowledge to enable her to continue education along general lines and not give conflicting advice. She would not of course be expected to have the in-depth diabetic knowledge of the clinical nurse specialist. She must be part of the team; without her considerable help the smooth efficient running of the outpatient department or day hospital could not take place.

Outpatient department nurses working in diabetic clinics and day hospitals need special training. New and inexperienced nurses plunged into a diabetic clinic require training and this slows the activity of the clinic and reduces its efficiency and detracts from the service. Managers must realize the importance of the nurse in maintaining continuity of care in the diabetic clinic. It is wrong to rotate nurses through specialized clinics producing an endless flow of new and untrained nurses. The clinics exist for the patients' benefit, not just to give the nurses experience.

Ward nurses require a basic training in diabetic care since diabetics may be present on any ward.

12.3.4 The clinical nurse specialist

(a) Diabetic ward sister

Like other sisters the diabetic ward sister must have extensive experience in general nursing and be an efficient manager. However, in addition she must be proficient in the skills of diabetic education and be an innovator. It is therefore necessary for her to have a specialized training in diabetes, teaching, and to be a keen member of the diabetic team. She must be involved in the formulation of policies for diabetic care within the hospital and indeed within the district. She would be expected to represent the views of the diabetic health care team on the management of diabetics and to persuade other service and ward managers to accept health care team policies on the management of diabetics no matter where lodged within the hospital.

(b) Diabetic liaison sister

The diabetic liaison sister should have a training equivalent to that of the ward sister. There should, however, be different emphasis. In addition to the general nursing qualification the diabetic liaison sister must obtain a community nursing qualification as she will be operating out of the hospital and in the community for part of her time. As for the ward sister she must have management experience and advanced training in diabetes and education.

The diabetic liaison sister must be prepared to work both within the hospital and within the community. In the hospital she will be required to work with the diabetic ward sister, the diabetic firm, and be prepared to follow up patients within the hospital and when they are discharged from the hospital into the community.

The diabetic liaison sister must be prepared to organize the outpatient/day hospital diabetic education sessions. This will involve close liaison with the dietitians and chiropodists.

The diabetic liaison sister should be available for consultation by practice-linked nurses and district nurses. She should also make herself available for giving patients advice at home either by means of home visits or by telephone calls. She should be prepared, under the supervision of the diabetologist, to convert patients to insulin therapy without the necessity of admitting the patient to hospital.

The diabetic liaison sister should be involved in training student and pupil nurses.

It will be seen that the post of diabetic liaison sister is, to say the least, a taxing one. It has been recommended that at least one diabetic liaison sister should be available per 50 000 of the population. This allows a ratio of one liaison sister to approximately 500 diabetic patients. Of these 60% may be totally managed in the community and 40% jointly managed in the community and in hospital (Royal College of Physicians of London and BDA, 1984).

12.4 TRAINING AND RESPONSIBILITIES

When considering the number of nurses and indeed all health care workers involved in diabetic care, it will be quickly appreciated that some form of organization and central education is essential. If confusion for the patient is to be avoided then it is essential for the diabetic health care team to speak with one voice. It is therefore important that the syllabus be clearly defined for the educators and those to be educated. The syllabus will obviously vary according to precisely which particular part of diabetic health service a nurse is working in but there will be a basic core of knowledge common to all.

Sections 12.4.1 and 12.4.2 indicate a syllabus for nurse training in addition to general nurse training during which some introduction to diabetes will be given.

12.4.1 Syllabus 1

For district/community nurses, practice linked nurses, outpatient/diabetic clinic/day hospital nurses and general ward nurses:

1. What is diabetes?
2. Establishing the diagnosis.
3. Short-term problems.
4. Long-term complications.
5. Treatment diet/oral hypoglycaemic agents/insulin.
6. Organization of diabetic care in the district.
7. Home monitoring – urine/blood.
8. What patients are taught. All videos, computer programs, slide or tape material and literature should be available to the nursing staff for small group and private study. It is essential for them to know what the patients are being taught.
9. Special course on ulcer/wound management in diabetics.
10. For practice linked nurses and outpatient nurses. The nurse conducted diabetic interview (see Chapter 6).

12.4.2 Syllabus 2

For the clinical nurse specialist:

1. Diabetes:
   (i) An overview of diabetes including aetiology, genetics, and epidemiology.

(ii) Making the diagnosis and initiating treatment.

(iii) Educating the diabetic.

(iv) The control of blood glucose concentration – treatment. This should include advanced experience in dietitics, the use of oral hypoglycaemic agents, and insulin delivery techniques. The specialist clinical nurse should be familiar with conventional insulin therapy, multiple injection techniques, and continuous subcutaneous infusion of insulin. She should be familiar with the methods of adjusting the dose of insulin and how to teach the patient to adjust their own insulin.

(v) Diabetic emergencies.

(vi) Follow-up. What is required in hospital and in the community. The role of the family and friends. Continued health education.

(vii) The organization of diabetic health care.

(viii) The long-term complications of diabetes.

(ix) The role of the nurse in diabetic care.

(x) The use of audit.

2. A course on education techniques.
3. Management.

12.4.3 Qualifications and post-graduate training required by nurses in diabetic care

1. District or community nurses:

   (i) General nursing qualification.

   (ii) District/community nursing qualification.

   (iii) In-service training in diabetes organized by the triumvirate (see text).

2. Practice linked nurses:

   (i) General nursing qualifications.

   (ii) In-service training organized by the triumvirate and the local family doctor.

   (iii) Special training in relations to the nurse follow-up interview (see Chapter 6).

3. Diabetic-clinic (outpatient department) nurse/day hospital nurse:

   (i) General nursing qualifications.

(ii) Inservice training in diabetes organized by the triumvirate.
(iii) In-service training in the diabetic clinic.

4. Specialist diabetic nurse. The following suggest an outline training:
   (i) General nursing qualifications.
   (ii) Extensive experience in general medicine.
   (iii) Experience to the seniority of sister:
      – Ward (diabetic ward sister).
      – Community nursing/district nursing sister.
   (iv) Management experience.
   (v) Advanced training in diabetes (Syllabus 2).
   (vi) Advanced training in education.

The English National Board Course (ENB No. 928) is held in various parts of the UK (in 1986 : Birmingham, Manchester and Portsmouth). It must be regarded as only the beginning of the training needed for a clinical nurse specialist which should be undertaken either before appointment or within the first 6 months of appointment.

As yet no higher qualification for the clinical nurse specialist in diabetes exists but this may not be long in coming as it is essential to recognize the expertise of the workers involved.

The responsibilities of the diabetic clinical nurse specialist may be summarized as follows:

1. Educational:
   (i) Patient education
   (ii) Staff education – ward nurses, outpatient/clinic/day hospital nurses, practice linked nurses, community nurses, dietitian, chiropodist, doctors.
2. Advisory:
   (i) Patient (24 hour service), after-care follow-up.
   (ii) Nurses.
   (iii) Doctors
3. Management and organization:
   (i) Ward
   (ii) OPD/clinic/day hospital/community.
4. Liaison : between hospital and district/community, patient and medical staff, medical and nursing staff.

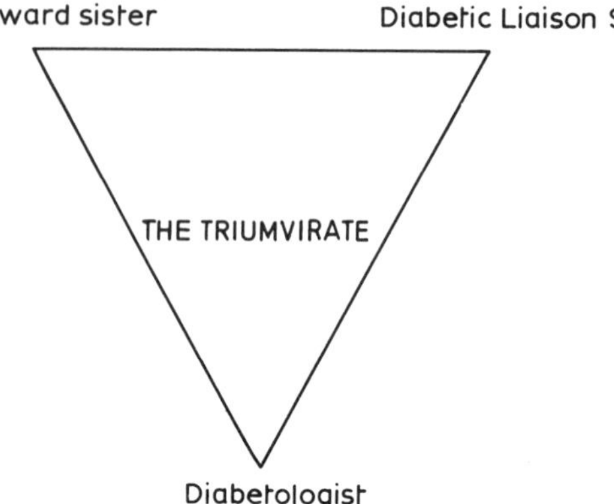

Figure 12.1 The triumvirate.

The diabetic ward sister, diabetic liaison sister, and the diabetologist constitute a **Triumvirate** (*Figure 12.1*) which can produce the driving force necessary to make the diabetic health care service successful.

12.5 ARE CLINICAL NURSE SPECIALISTS IN DIABETES EFFECTIVE AND COST EFFECTIVE?

Such a question is easy to formulate but quantifying the answer is difficult. Most diabetologists know in their hearts that the clinical nurse specialists are effective in improving diabetic care. However, this subjective response is not enough when requesting resources to fund a post.

All health services have finite resources and there will be competitive bids for a share of the financial cake. Such a bid must be carefully planned (see section 12.10) and contain information indicating in what way a clinical nurse specialist is likely to be effective in improving diabetic care and how this will be cost effective.

That clinical nurse specialists can be effective in improving the standard of diabetic care has been shown in the Birmingham Children's Clinic where the standard of glycaemic control as indicated by HbA_1 values, improved from 13.1% before the introduction of the nurse to 11.4% after the introduction of the clinical nurse specialist. (Rayner, 1984).

Table 12.1 The effect of introducing clinical nurse specialists

	Before	*After*
Admission rate per 1000 patients per year	670	130
DKA per 1000 patients per year	38.8	8.6
Amputations per 1000 patients per year	13.3	6.72
Days in hospital per 1000 patients per year	5.6	0.82

In another study, after the introduction of an open 24 hour service staffed by specialist diabetic nurses, there was considerable reduction (to one fifth) in the admisison rate, the admission rate for diabetic ketoacidosis, and length of stay in hospital. Even more dramatically the amputation rate was halved (Davidson, 1983) (*Table 12.1*).

In Poole General Hospital the appointment of a second clinical nurse specialist would cost £10 816 but would save 520 bed days per annum equivalent to a cost of £66 000 (1986).

It may therefore be concluded that the introduction of clinical nurse specialists is both effective in improving the standards of care and proves very cost effective.

12.6 PLANNING FOR SUCCESS

The application for resources for a diabetic clinical nurse specialist should take into account that resources are finite. Any application for a share of resources must be planned and set out in such a way as to convince management of the need and to justify the increase in expenditure. Any material saving strongly supports the application in these impoverished times. It is suggested that the following planning profile will aid such an application.

1. Assess the need. Include a priority rating and some indication of the implications for the rest of the service as a whole. This might include the possibility of reducing the number of beds used for converting diabetics to insulin therapy in hospital leaving them available for other purposes.
2. Plan of operation. The modus operandi of the clinical nurse specialist should be clearly set out. A job description should be prepared but this should allow flexibility to enable the individual to change, develop and evolve the service.

3. A case of need should be prepared to include all anticipated recurring and non-recurring costs. For instance, secretarial help, accommodation, uniform travel costs and equipment might be included. It is important to be realistic and not over ambitious. Clearly indicate that the development could be implemented on a phased basis.
4. The expected advantages in terms of improved standards of care resulting from the introduction of a clinical nurse specialist should be clearly stated.
5. A simple cost benefit analysis should be attempted to demonstrate the potential savings from the introduction of a clinical nurse specialist.
6. A paper based on (1) – (5) above should be prepared and submitted.
7. Unashamed lobbying of all and sundry should then take place!

12.7 IMPLEMENTATION

Once a clinical nurse specialist has been appointed it is important to ensure that the successful candidate is integrated into the health care team both in the hospital and in the community. It is essential to avoid isolation and maintain her managerial contacts. It is important to establish the case load and to advise on and review the work done. Any job description will need modifying in the light of developments and experience, and flexibility must be maintained.

The service will require careful monitoring and evaluation. Evaluation should take place at an agreed date. This should be to review progress over a standard period of time and to assess the service provided as perceived by nurses, doctors, and above all the patients. In addition to this the time spent on clinical work, education, administration, and travelling should be assessed.

12.8 CONCLUSION

The functions served by nursing are summarized in a statement from the code of ethics of the International Council of Nurses :

> 'Nurses minister to the sick, assume responsibility for creating a physical, social and spiritual environment which will be conducive to recovery, and stress the prevention of illness and promo-

> tion of health by teaching and example. They render health service to the individual, the family and the community, and co-ordinate their services with members of other health professions. Service to mankind is the primary function of nurses and the reason for the existence of the nursing profession. Need for nursing service is universal. Professional nursing service is therefore unrestricted by considerations of nationality, race, colour, political or social status.'

This statement summarizes precisely the role of the nurse in diabetic care.

REFERENCES AND FURTHER READING

Connor, H. (1984) Diabetic management and education: cost and benefits. In *Diabetes Education* (eds. A.K. Baksi, D.W. Hyde, and G. Giles), John Wiley, Chichester, pp. 1–20.

Davidson, J.K. (1983) *The Grady Memorial Hospital Diabetes Unit Ambulatory Care Programme.* Excerpta Medica International Congress Series No. 624, pp. 286–97.

Diabetes Education Study Group of the European Association for the Study of Diabetes. *Teaching Centre List for Health Care Team Visitors.* (Secretary : Professor M. Berger, 2, Med. Universitatsklinik, 5 Mooren Strasse D4, Dusseldorf).

Rayner, P.H.W. (1984) Home care unit for diabetic children. *Practical Diabetes*, **1**, 5.

Royal College of Physicians of London Committee on Endocrinology and Diabetes Mellitus and British Diabetic Association Report (1984). *The provision of medical care for adult diabetic patients in the United Kingdom.*

· Thirteen ·

The organization of diabetic health care

13.1 INTRODUCTION

There are a large number of workers in diabetic health care:

1. Primary health care:
   (i) The patient and relatives/friends.
   (ii) The family doctors.
   (iii) Practice linked nurses, district nurses.
   (iv) Practice staff – secretaries, receptionists.
   (v) Chiropodists.
   (vi) Dietitians.
   (vii) Ophthalmic medical practitioners and ophthalmic opticians.
   (viii) Pharmacists.
2. Secondary health care:
   (i) Doctors: generalist/specialist.
   (ii) Nurses.
   (iii) Dietitians.
   (iv) Chiropodists.
   (v) Medical records – receptionists, clerks, secretaries, porters.
   (vi) Pharmacists.
   (vii) Laboratory staff.
   (viii) Radiographers (X-ray department staff).
   (ix) Administrators.
   (x) Telephonists.

Not forgetting the numerous other workers such as those who work in the maintenance department, electricians, etc. who beaver away quietly in the background to keep a busy district general hospital running. The list is no doubt incomplete and I will be criticized for missing out important members of the service (doctors' spouses for instance!) However, it is intended to indicate the large number of workers involved. No matter how important you consider your part to be in the health care service you cannot function properly without the work of others.

The division of the health services into primary and secondary health care is a useful descriptive device but in practice it may be counter-productive if boundaries are created. This is particularly a problem in medical and nursing areas. The family doctor working in the community may be regarded as a less skilled worker by the arrogant hospital doctor. The family doctor bridles at any 'interference' by the hospital-based doctor. Animosity may exist between hospital ophthalmic services and ophthalmic opticians working in a district. Hopefully, in the future this antagonism will be broken down.

The separation of 'hospital' and 'community' nursing services is a good example of professional restrictive practice. A rigid adherence to job description and job demarcation can only be detrimental to the service. A senior nursing administrator once suggested to me that 'a health visitor may advise and explain but may not do, and a community nurse may do but may not advise'!

A failure to recognize that we are all but small cogs in the health care machine produces disharmony, inefficiency, and a poor service for the patient. The *raison d'être* for our existence is to provide health care, and not to provide jobs for the boys! We should strive to improve the service in every way and recognize the importance and worth of every member of the health care team. Any boundaries created between primary and secondary health care must be broken down and an integrated service developed.

The realization that health care cannot be compartmentalized is perhaps the first of many stages in the evolution of health care. It is difficult to change attitudes and open minds to new ideas. This tends to be the case with people in rigid patterns of management who are not at the sharp end of health care. However, with gentle persuasion and explanation and a great deal of persistence this can be done. An integrated service will not just happen. It will come about only by organization, extra effort, extra input, and determination to change hard and ingrained attitudes, particularly of doctors and nursing staff.

In any health care system, if one section fails to do its job properly then another section will be forced to take extra work. This eventually leads to overload in certain sections of the service with a breakdown and failure of the service . . . a medical 'domino effect'. An example of the misuse of skills in secondary health care is seen when patients with diabetes are referred to ophthalmologists for **screening** examinations. The ophthalmologist has specialskills and special training which could be more usefully employed. It is the responsibility of primary health care and the diabetologist to organize the service in such a way that **screening** can take place and a **selection** of patients requiring either an opinion or treatment be presented to the ophthalmologist. Only by doing this will his special skills be properly utilized (Chapter 7).

There should be an interchange of skills between primary and secondary health care. The diabetologist should be available to make house calls (domiciliary visits) at the request of a primary health care doctor. Similarly he should be available on the telephone to discuss patients and problems and give advice when it is sought. The primary health care doctor should have free access to certain relevant hospital facilities and be free to attend the wards in the hospital for joint discussion and consultation. It is my experience that few primary health care doctors avail themselves of this facility simply because they are too busy and are quite happy to leave the management of the diabetic in hospital to the hospital-based team. He should play a part in secondary health care as a clinical assistant.

The specialist nurse (e.g. diabetic liaison sister) should move freely between community and hospital: the specialist nurse ideally attends all ward rounds and is involved in outpatient work and teaching sessions. She visits patients, teaches, converts patients to insulin therapy in the home and acts as a trouble shooter in the community. (see Chapter 12).

The dietitian may under certain circumstances also provide a domiciliary service where the patient is not able to travel into the hospital.

A community chiropody service is essential since the patients requiring the most chiropody are elderly (Chapter 11).

13.2 AREAS OF RESPONSIBILITY

When considering 'who should be doing what' it is convenient to look at three areas of responsibility:

1. The responsibilities of the patient.
2. Responsibilities of primary health care.
3. Responsibilities of secondary health care.

13.2.1 The responsibilities of the patient

These may be set out as follows:

1. To manage his/her own diabetic state.
2. To acquire the necessary knowledge and practical skills to achieve (1) above.
3. To actively seek follow-up for eye care, foot care, blood pressure measurement, interval blood sugar and HbA1 measurements and to expect this to be provided by the diabetic health care team.
4. To expect that certain specialist services will be made available to the diabetic should he/she need them.

13.2.2 Responsibilities of primary health care

These may be set out as follows:

1. To maintain a high index of suspicion in order to detect diabetes in an early stage and to reach an early diagnosis.
2. To confirm the diagnosis of diabetes mellitus to WHO criteria.
3. To initiate treatment (first aid) and start the educational process. The family doctor is expected at this stage to act as a family doctor and be reassuring and sympathetic.
4. To refer patients to an education session or provide it.
5. To modify treatment to achieve satisfactory standards of control.
6. To provide routine follow up for diabetics (6 months maximum interval) to assess the standard of glycaemic control (interval blood sugar and HbA1), the presence of abnormal renal function (albuminuria and serum creatinine), the maintenance of normal body weight, and to detect the presence of raised blood pressure or long-term complications of diabetes.
7. To refer patients to secondary health care when the need arises.
8. To provide an efficient appointment system which will detect patients who fail to attend. A recall system is essential.
9. To provide a domiciliary service for the elderly.

10. To organize practice linked nurses and community nurses to provide help for those patients who need it.
11. To liaise with the specialist diabetic nurse and with the hospital based health care team.

13.2.3 Responsibilities of secondary health care

The specialist in diabetes must accept the role of leader. He should collect demographic data on the district served by his hospital, make projections into the future to assess future needs, and then define clearly what is required of the diabetic service. He should review the diabetic service and be responsible for righting any deficiencies and improving the efficiency of the service.

The hospital based services must provide the following:

1. Diabetic education facilities.
2. Initial review and assessment.
3. Laboratory services.
4. Special follow-up clinics for special problems:
   (i) Retinal.
   (ii) Renal.
   (iii) Peripheral vascular disease.
   (iv) Routine follow-up of insulin treated diabetics where necessary and for the follow-up of patients with special problems.
5. Chiropody service.
6. Dietitian service.
7. The hospital based service must provide suitable monitoring and audit facilities, preferably computer based, for the whole district.

It is important that the influence of the diabetic service should spread out beyond the bounds of the hospital. It should extend into primary health care in the spirit of partnership. The specialist in diabetes must be prepared to go out into the community, talk to family doctors, district nurses, practice linked nurses and other workers in order to inform them of the ways in which the service works and at the same time make them feel that they are part of an efficient team providing a necessary service. The interchange of information provides the essential feedback necessary for corrective measures to be taken to improve the service as a whole.

Secondary health care must include educational facilities not only for patients but also for all workers whether in primary or secondary health care and to provide regular update sessions. It must be remembered that the health care worker population is not a static one. There is a constant movement with juniors coming in and more experienced workers retiring. A failure to provide regular update sessions will result in eventual chaos.

Educational groups for which secondary health care must take some responsibility are:

1. Hospital doctors – regular clinical meetings within the hospital.
2. Family doctor educational sessions should be organized by the specialist in diabetes in consulation with local family doctors. Regular communications detailing changes or problems within the service must be sent to all doctors. A word processor is valuable in this respect. This allows personalized letters to be sent to all doctors within the district without overloading hospital secretarial facilities.
3. Where ophthalmic opticians provide a service, annual meetings are necessary to provide up-to-date information, maintain momentum, and acquire feedback.
4. Nursing staff. Regular meetings must be arranged to update nurses since there is a high turnover rate amongst nursing staff. This is particularly important with regard to nurses working within the community.
5. Other small groups such as chiropodists, dietitians, pharmacy workers and laboratory workers usually have their own societies and meetings. It is possible from time to time to incorporate into one of these sessions details of the diabetic health care service, its problems, its solutions, and its aspirations. This type of effort is valuable in that it helps to make the health care service work smoothly and efficiently, and at the same time boost the morale of workers. They no longer feel that they are a forgotten group of workers providing a service which is unsung and unthanked.
6. It is also worth while very occasionally arranging meetings for medical secretaries and receptionists etc. from the community for similar reasons to those stated above.

13.3 THE COMMUNITY CARE SERVICE FOR DIABETICS IN THE POOLE AREA. A CASE STUDY FOR DIABETES HEALTH CARE

To illustrate that what has been said is not pure theory but has been put into practice, a description of the present situation in Poole will follow. It is important to realize that the service is not a static one but is evolving all the time. It is not intended to suggest that this is the only way ahead for diabetic care. It serves to indicate how one area with a typical age/sex structure within the United Kingdom (Gatling *et al.*, 1985) has attempted to cope with the problem of diabetic care in a rapidly growing community. It has been suggested that Poole is 'atypical' and that 'the service would be unsuitable for other areas'. This may be so, but I wonder how atypical of the United Kingdom Poole really is. The most vociferous (particularly in terms of the printed word) are those excellent specialists from medical school based clinics. These are often situated in the centre of large conurbations. These have their own problems. The standard of primary health care may be poor, cities are often the centre of social deprivation and often contain large racial minorities. I think perhaps that this situation is atypical and that when many physicians take the opportunity of looking at their own demographic data they will realize that their situation approximates more closely to Poole than to the inner city situation.

13.3.1 Introduction

In 1970 a review of the population for the Eastern Sector of the East Dorset Health Authority revealed a frightening growth rate (*Table 13.1*). In addition to this a review of the diabetic service showed:

Table 13.1 Poole is the sixth fastest growing town in the UK

	1951	*1961*	*1971*	*1981*	*1991*	*2001*
Eastern sector	160	183	188	182	177	171
Western sector (Poole)	140	160	195	228	260	292
Total (1000)	307	343	383	410	437	463

By 1991 East Dorset will be the largest Health Care District in Wessex.

1. Less than 50% of the expected number of diabetics attended or had attended the diabetic clinic.
2. The only contribution to diabetic care made by the hospital was a single overcrowded diabetic clinic held once per week.
3. Waiting times in the clinic were long.
4. There was no organized co-operation between primary and secondary health care.
5. The laboratory services were overstressed on one day of the week with little or no use of the laboratory service by diabetics on other days of the week.

Clearly, with the projected population growth the current service as organized would break down, and a dramatic reorganization was necessary to provide a service in the foreseeable future.

In 1971 the Community Care Service was set up at a joint meeting of primary and secondary health care doctors. At this meeting 92% of all patients attending the Diabetic Clinic at that time were represented by his or her family doctor, or a partner. One hundred and five family doctors attended this meeting (Hill, 1976a).

At this meeting a decision was made to develop a Community Care Service. This was to be a shared care system of diabetic care, a partnership between primary health care on the one hand and secondary health care on the other. To this end a working party was set up consisting of prominent local family doctors (which included the Clinical Tutor and Diabetic Clinic Assistant) and the Consultant in charge of the Diabetic Clinic at Poole General Hospital. The working party organized the following:

1. Postgraduate training in diabetes to involve family doctors, practice linked nurses, district nurses, and practice administration staff.
2. Design and develop a Co-operation Booklet which would be a means of communication between family doctors, hospital doctors, nurses, and the patient. It would also form the basis of a clinical record and be part of the education programme for patient and health care workers in the scheme.
3. In conjunction with the department of biochemistry the 2 hour interval blood sugar system was introduced. In this system patients attend the laboratory 2 hours after a meal for an interval blood sugar on any day of the week, Monday to Friday. They may attend at any time between 9 a.m. and 4.30 p.m. There is no

waiting and 97% of patients are in and out of the laboratory within 20 minutes.

The main concept behind the Community Care Service is that of regarding the patient as the most important person in the health care team looking after the diabetic. To this end the Community Care Service attempts to:

1. Provide the diabetic with theoretical knowledge and practical skills to enable him or her to look after him or herself.
2. To provide support in the community at the family doctor/district nurse level.
3. To provide specialist advice and services as follows (Hill, 1976b; 1979; Hill and Upton, 1981):
   (i) Diabetic education sessions. Continued diabetic education.
   (ii) Open dietitian service.
   (iii) Chiropody service.
   (iv) Full clinical and laboratory assessment.
   (v) Diabetic review clinic.
   (vi) Routine follow-up in the diabetic clinic.
   (vii) Primary health care screening programme for diabetic eye disease and joint retinal clinic.
   (viii) The specialist services of a diabetic liaison sister.
4. To provide a laboratory open service to family doctors.
5. To provide liaison between primary and secondary health care.

13.3.2 The Community Care Service in practice, 1986

(a) Diagnosis in primary health care

Apart from emergency cases the majority of diabetics are diagnosed by the general practitioner. No patient is referred to the hospital until a diagnosis has been established on WHO criteria (see section 1.3).

Once the diagnosis has been established the patient is reassured and given first aid advice. A standard letter of introduction to the diabetic education session is provided for all family doctors to use (*Figure 13.1*).

The usual letter of referral to the diabetic review clinic is either sent by post or given to the patient to bring to the diabetic education session. The patients first contact with secondary health care is at this session and takes place within 6 days of establishing the diagnosis.

Figure 13.1 ►

Poole General Hospital
Longfleet Road
Poole, Dorset
Poole 675100 Extension 2399
DEPARTMENT OF DIABETES

G.P. Stamp:

Date:

Dear Patient,

If your diabetes is newly diagnosed you will no doubt be anxious about the future. Let us reassure you right away that with proper care and treatment you will be able to live a full and normal life. You may feel better than your non-diabetic friends! Even if you have had diabetes for some time you may be apprehensive about what sort of service we will provide. You will be pleased to hear that you have moved to a district which makes a special effort to care for those with diabetes.

The Community Care Service for Diabetes in the Poole area was formed in 1971. It comprises a team of workers helping **you** to look after **yourself** and manage **your** diabetes. **REMEMBER** that the most important person in the Health Care Team looking after the diabetic is **you.**

Your first introduction to the service has already taken place when you consulted your own family doctor. Your next contact with the service will be at the Diabetic Education Session.

The Diabetic Education Session takes place on Friday afternoons in the Green Clinic, Poole General Hospital. You should attend **Friday next at 1.45 p.m. prompt.** You must expect to be there all afternoon. There you will be given an introduction to diabetes, advice on diet, information about the Community Care Service, and taught many other things relating to diabetes. The Education Session is run by the Diabetic Liaison Sister and the Dietitian. The session is informal and friendly and you will be given plenty of time to ask questions. You will not see a doctor on this occasion unless there is some urgent need when this will be arranged by the Diabetic Liaison Sister.

Before coming to the Diabetic Education Session may we offer this simple advice on your diet:

Dont's	**Do's**
DO NOT add sugar to any drink or food.	SUGAR FREE sweeteners may be used if necessary.
AVOID all sweetened drinks, jams, marmalade, honey.	LOW calorie or sugar free drinks and sugar free preserves may be used.
DO NOT eat sugary puddings or desserts, tinned fruit in syrup, tinned milk puddings or jellies.	INSTEAD have fresh or stewed fruit, using a sugar free sweetener if necessary or fruit tinned without sugar.
AVOID all sweet biscuits, cakes, sweets, chocolate and diabetic alternatives.	BUT if you are hungry between meals have a piece of fruit.
DO NOT eat low-fibre, starchy foods: white bread and flour, low fibre crisp breads, biscuits and breakfast cereals, white pasta and rice.	INSTEAD have fibre-rich foods: wholemeal bread and flour, high fibre crispbreads, biscuits and breakfast cereals, wholemeal pasta and brown rice, jacket potatoes and vegetables especially peas and beans.

Your meals can be planned in your normal way – providing you have cut out the sugar and refined foods, as this will start to bring your diabetes under control.

If you are also overweight, you should reduce the amount of fat you eat by using less butter, margarine, oil, lard, dripping and cheese. **This is stop-gap advice for you to follow until you see the dietitian who will plan a personal diet with you.**

REMEMBER

Look forward to a healthier life!
Attend the next Diabetic Education Session on Friday next at
1.45 p.m. the Green Clinic, Poole General Hospital.
Test your urine once daily or as instructed by your doctor.
Take the simple advice given above.

We look forward to meeting you.

Yours sincerely,

R.D. HILL, FRCP
Consultant Physician

All patients whether newly diagnosed or diabetics new to the area are asked to attend the diabetic education session, and it is by this route that patients are referred on further to the diabetic review clinic and gain entry to the scheme.

(b) Diabetic education service

Teaching in the diabetic education session is carried out on the basis of group teaching, small group teaching, and individual tuition. The sessions are conducted by the diabetic liaison sister, dietitians and chiropodists. Eight to twelve patients plus their relatives are seen at any one session.

Session 1:

2.00 p.m. *Introduction to Diabetes* (tape/slide programme).
2.30 p.m. *Introduction to Diet* (tape/slide programme).
3.00 p.m. *Tea*
3.15 p.m. *Dietary Assessment* Urine testing.

Session 2:

2.00 p.m. *Question and answer.*
2.10 p.m. *Co-operation Book.*
2.30 p.m. *Urine testing revisions.*
2.40 p.m. *Foot Care* (tape/slide programme).
3.00 p.m. *Tea.*
3.15 p.m. *Chiropody assessment*
Dietitian.
Counselling.
Diabetic Review Clinic Appointment.

The diabetic liaison sister also conducts further education sessions on home blood glucose monitoring (meter clinics). Continued education is also carried out by the chiropodist, the dietitian, the doctors in the diabetic clinic and the doctors in primary health care at every session where the patient meets members of the health care team.

Any patient requiring urgent attention when attending the diabetic education session (e.g. with ketonuria or who feels ill or has some diabetic complication) is seen by a doctor at the diabetic education session and an assessment made. Otherwise the patient continues under the care of the family doctor on a diet with or without oral hypoglycaemic agents. The patient is asked to test the urine once per day at different times throughout the day and the results are recorded. When the patient attends the diabetic review clinic he will have already been taking a diet with or without oral hypoglycaemic agents, will have urine tests available to show the doctor, and will in most cases have an interval blood sugar and haemoglobin A1 (at least one estimation). In addition to this a weight at the start of dietary treatment will be available for comparison with a weight at the clinic. Before patients attend the diabetic review clinic they are asked to attend for routine investigations, i.e. electrocardiogram (ECG), interval blood sugar (IBS), haemoglobin A1 (HbA1), serum creatinine, liver function tests, cholesterol and triglycerides.

(c) Diabetic review clinic

Diabetic review clinic initial appointment (7–8 patients). This clinic is held on Monday afternoons between 1.30 p.m. and 6 p.m. Seven or eight newly diagnosed diabetics or diabetics new to the area have a full assessment at this clinic. A full history is taken and a complete clinical examination made. The data are recorded in the diabetic clinic notes. Examination includes distant visual acuity measurement, dilatation of the pupils, and examination of the eyes. A review of the history, clinical examination, the routine investigations, and the standard of control achieved is undertaken and adjustment made to the treatment as is necessary. Education is continued.

Patients are then asked to return to the diabetic review clinic for a follow-up appointment, usually in 1–3 months.

Diabetic review clinic follow-up appointment (eight patients). All patients are seen by the diabetologist:

1. To review the standard of control achieved.
2. To solve any problems that are developing.
3. To continue education.

By the time the patient attends for the second appointment the patient, with the aid of the family doctor, has achieved the maximum control possible with diet alone or diet together with oral hypoglycaemic agents. At this session patients are classified into various groups:

Group 1. Controlled on diet alone (interval blood sugar 3–7 mmol/1, haemoglobin A1 8.5% or less) – upper limit of normal in this laboratory).

Group 2. Controlled on diet plus oral hypoglycaemic agent (glibenclamide maximum dose 20 mg per day, gliclazide maximum dose 320 mg per day, or equivalent sulphonylurea or metformin in a few selected cases of obesity) (interval blood sugar 3–7 mmol/1, haemoglobin A1 8.5% or less).

Group 3. Not controlled with diet or oral hypoglycaemic agent.

Group 4. Insulin-treated diabetics.

Groups 1 and 2 are transferred to general practice for routine follow-up. They are given a full explanation of what this means. They are also given a small booklet entitled *Transferred to GP's care* (*Table 3.1*) and are then shown a brief slide/tape film which reiterates all that they have been told and reinforces the importance of continued care.

Group 3 diabetics are transferred to insulin treatment either at home with the help of the diabetic liaison sister (depending on geographical location and diabetic liaison sister's workload) or in hospital. After transfer to insulin treatment patients are followed up in the routine diabetic clinic (Friday afternoon).

The standard of control achieved by group 4 patients is assessed. Adjustments are made and they are then transferred to the routine diabetic clinic for follow-up.

Patients with associated long-term complications of diabetes are either followed up at routine diabetic clinic or at one of the special diabetic clinics outlined below.

(d) Routine diabetic clinic (Friday afternoon)

This clinic caters mainly for insulin treated diabetics and diabetics with a problem (e.g. control or long-term complications). It is staffed by four doctors (one consultant, two clinical assistants, and one registrar); 70–80 patients are seen.

The chiropodist service and the diabetic education session run concurrently with the routine diabetic clinic.

There is also a British Diabetic Association Stand, manned by volunteers, giving information and selling various items of equipment and the publications of the British Diabetic Association.

(e) Medical outpatients

Patients with added non-diabetic complications (such as asthma or polymyalgia etc.) are seen in the routine medical outpatients follow-up clinic on Thursday afternoons, staffed by two doctors. Thirty-six patients are seen.

(f) Diabetic eye disease

A confidential enquiry (Hill, unpublished) indicated that many family doctors were unhappy about their ability to examine the eye to the standard required for screening for diabetic eye disease. Ophthalmic medical practitioners and ophthalmic opticians were asked to co-operate in the development of a screening programme for diabetic eye disease. They agreed to accept the definitions of diabetic eye disease and to carry out documentation and coding. This forms the basis of the primary health care screening programme for diabetic eye disease (see Chapter 7; also Hill, 1981).

(g) Joint retinal clinic

All patients with diabetic eye disease are assessed by the diabetologist. Patients requiring an ophthalmological opinion, i.e. if the exact diagnosis is in doubt, or those requiring photocoagulation, are referred to the joint retinal clinic. Otherwise such patients are followed up in the routine diabetic clinic.

The joint retinal clinic is held on Tuesday morning. It is a joint consultative clinic conducted by a consultant ophthalmic surgeon, and a diabetologist. A routine diagnostic and follow-up clinic is held on alternate Tuesdays, alternating with a treatment (xenon arc) clinic. Argon laser therapy is carried out by the ophthalmic surgeon at the Royal Victoria Eye Hospital, Westbourne, on Wednesday afternoons when required; 12–16 patients are seen at the diagnostic and follow-up clinic, approximately four patients at any one time are seen in the treatment clinic.

(h) Diabetic nephropathy clinic (DNC)

Patients with diabetic nephropathy are followed up at a special clinic held on Tuesday mornings which alternates with the joint retinal clinic. Diabetic patients who satisfy one or more of the following criteria are followed up in this clinic:

1. Early morning urine (EMU) albumin/creatinine ratio 3.5 or more.
2. Overnight albumin excretion rate (AER) of 30 μg/min or more.

3. Intermittent proteinuria (Albustix + (30 mg%) or greater)
4. Persistent proteinuria (Albustix + (30 mg%) or greater).
5. Serum creatinine 150 μmol/1. or more.

Patients for dialysis and transplantation are assessed at a monthly clinic by a visiting physician from the regional dialysis and transplant unit.

(i) Diabetics living in outlying areas

Patients living at a distance from Poole General Hospital in the Blandford area (18 miles (30 km) distant) are seen at the Blandford Community Hospital by the diabetologist in a general medical outpatient clinic (held every 2 weeks) and are routinely followed up by a clinical assistant, running a diabetic clinic once per month.

(j) The role of the diabetic liaison sister

1. Outpatient education sessions.
2. Stabilization and education of diabetics requiring insulin treatment at home (see Section 3.3 and Chapter 12).
3. Follow-up of various patients in the home.
4. Liaison between community and hospital staff.

The diabetic liaison sister has also been instrumental in the development of the various education systems used within the service.

(k) The diabetic ward staff

Apart from the routine management of in-patients, the management of diabetic problems and the education of diabetic patients in the ward is the special province of the ward sister. She has developed various visual aids and methods of teaching diabetics when in the ward (see section 3.3 and Chapter 12).

(l) Role of the family doctor in the community care service for diabetics in the Poole area

Apart from maintaining a high index of suspicion with regard to the diagnosis of diabetes, family doctors are asked to not only make the initial diagnosis but to confirm this biochemically and initiate early treatment. To aid them in their efforts, the above services have been developed. In particular the biochemistry department provides open access to the family doctor. They are also asked to routinely follow-

Table 13.2 Standards of control

Place of follow-up	%	*IBS* (mmol/l)	*HbA1* (%)
Poole General Hospital Diabetic Clinic	37	9.6*	9.3*
Family doctor	63	8.9*	8.8**

Significant difference * P = 0.01; ** P = 0.001.

up certain diabetics with regular review of standard of control achieved and examination to detect long-term complications (see *Table 3.1*).

The efficiency of GP follow-up is difficult to evaluate. The standards of glycaemic control achieved by family doctors in the scheme have been assessed (Gatling, MD Thesis, University of Southampton, 1986) (*Table 13.2*).

It will be seen that 63% of patients are now routinely followed up by their family doctors. The standard of care in terms of IBS and HbA1 are better in the family doctor group and this is in keeping with the policy of transferring well controlled and uncomplicated patients to GP care.

Clinical impressions are always dangerous. However, we do have the hard fact that no patient has been referred to the diabetic review clinic, diabetic clinic, medical outpatients or joint retinal clinic, with disease related to neglect of a patient in primary health care. In addition to this, we have had no unavoidable case of ketoacidosis for some years and no episode of diabetic coma.

Without the full co-operation of the family doctors in the area, the service would be impossible. The organization of the Diabetic Service within general practice is entirely a matter for the general practice concerned. Most family doctors in the area see their own diabetics. However, some practices run ‘mini clinics’ in which all diabetics within the practice are seen on a set day by one doctor specifically interested in diabetes. This has been tried in some practices and abandoned because of the problem of doctors going on holiday and other doctors not knowing anything about the patients when problems arise. Below, four family doctors give thumbnail sketches of their own practice organization of diabetic care. This may be of some help to those attempting to perform a similar exercise. Two examples are from market town/semi rural practices, and two examples are given from typical urban practice.

MARKET TOWN/RURAL PRACTICES

Practice A

Practice population – 12 000
Number of principals – Five plus one trainee (list size 2400)
Number of premises – one (with Community Hospital and GP beds).
Age/sex structure of population – that of UK.
Social class structure – a good spread between social classes II, III and IV.
Type of practice – semi-rural and rural (small market town 18 miles (30 km) distance from Poole General Hospital).
Number of diabetics in practice – 150 identified by repeat prescriptions, surgery attendance, and the Poole Diabetic Register. No disease register maintained in the practice.

Diabetic management in practice – a routine diabetic follow-up clinic is held monthly. Patients are referred from colleagues in the practice. Approximately 60 patients are followed up on a regular basis, the remainder being followed up either in the hospital diabetic clinic or by other colleagues in the practice. Routine diabetic follow-up clinic is held at the local community hospital; the sister in charge of outpatients runs the clinic.

Other principals in the practice see certain diabetics in routine surgery visits and not in an organized diabetic follow-up session.

Organization of practice diabetic clinic – the sister in charge organizes documentation (Poole Diabetic Clinic Notes), urine testing, height and weight and visual acuity. A dietitian visits. A doctor takes further history, completes documentation and any examination necessary. Time allowed for follow-up – 15 minutes with the doctor. Follow-up interval – 1–12 months. Follow-up appointments are sent to the patient 4 weeks before the appointment. A very low failure to attend rate has been achieved.

Advantages – Continuity of care. A spirit of co-operation with a regular enhancement of basic learning. Doctors consider that by routine follow-up the time actually spent solving problems is reduced as are unnecessary visits.

Practice B

Practice population – 13 500
Number of principals – Six plus one trainee.
Number of surgeries – One (with community hospital and GP beds).
Age/sex structure of the population – that of the UK.
Social class structure spread between social classes, II, III and IV.
Type of practice – small market town, semi-rural/rural, 7 miles (11 km) distance from Poole General Hospital.
Number of diabetics in practice – 137, identified by repeat prescriptions, Poole Diabetic Register, and surgery attendance. The practice is a dispensing practice with three dispensers. Follow-up discipline is maintained on the basis of no attendance for follow-up equals no repeat prescription.

Diabetic management in practice – There is no formal diabetic clinic. This was a conscious practice decision. The patient lists in this practice are highly personalized and each partner sees his own patients on a regular basis. Patients attend the practice for haemoglobin A1 and interval blood sugar (blood taken by nurse). Specimens are sent to Poole General Hospital laboratory. The results are available when patients attend for follow-up. The practice nurse also tests urine, weighs the patient, and checks blood pressures. Visual acuities when required are usually measured by the doctor. The doctor undertakes routine follow-up of diabetic patients on a 3–12 montly basis. Full examination is made on an annual or bi-annual review.

Author's note – The principals in this practice are highly qualified and provide an excellent personalized service. There is considerable interpartner referral for specific problems. Although no specific diabetic clinic is maintained in the practice, the personal approach to the patients has produced a highly efficient follow-up service.

URBAN PRACTICES

Practice C

Practice population – 8200.
Number of principals – 3½ (list size 2546).
Number of surgeries (health centre) – 1.
Age/sex structure – that of the UK.

Social class structure – predominantly III and IV.
Type of practice – urban.
Number of diabetics – 109 identified by repeat prescriptions, surgery attendance, the Poole Diabetic Register, and the Practice Disease Register (universal index cards).

Diabetic management in practice – Patients attend Poole General Hospital for a 2-hour interval blood sugar and HbA1 2 weeks before appointment. Reports are received in the practice after an interval of approximately 1 week.

Diabetic clinics are held on Tuesday mornings every 2 months. These are run by the practice nurse and patients see their own doctor.

The practice nurse takes a history and undertakes necessary documentation (patients' Co-operation Book). She weighs the patient, tests the urine, and makes an annual assessment of blood pressure and distant visual acuity. Mydriatics are used when the eyes are examined by the doctor.

The doctor sees the patient and reviews the nurse's findings. He reviews the patient's own monitoring and the information in the Co-operation Book. Examination as required is made.

The consultation time with the nurse is approximately 7 minutes and a similar time is spent with the doctor.

It has been found in practice that an improved through put of patients has been achieved by alternating diabetic patients with non-diabetic patients. This means that non-diabetic patients are slotted in to the diabetic clinic but this does not appear to cause any problems.

Follow-up appointments are sent by receptionist/secretary who also arranges the recall of non-attenders. Persistent non-attenders are sometimes visited by the health visitors.

Practice D

Practice population – 135 000
Number of principals – 7 (plus trainee) (list size 2167).
Number of surgeries – 1.
Age/sex structure – that of UK.
Social class structure – distribution to III and IV.
Type of practice – urban.
Number of diabetics – 130 identified from repeat prescriptions,

surgery attendances, and Poole Diabetic Register. Fifty per cent are followed up in the practice diabetic clinic and 50% followed up in hospital diabetic clinic.

Diabetic management in practice – An organized diabetic clinic was first set up by a GP trainee as part of her project (she now works as a clinical assistant in Poole General Hospital diabetic clinic). It was a practice decision that one doctor should look after all diabetic patients in practice. Patients attend the surgery nurse for a 2 hour interval blood sugar and HbA1 2 weeks before each visit. Electrolytes, urea, creatinine, measured annually. The practice nurse measures patient's weight, blood pressure, distant visual acuity, and tests urine. Information is recorded in patient's notes and Co-operation Book. The doctor in the practice diabetic clinic checks the standard of control achieved on the basis of HbA1, interval blood sugar and the patient's own monitoring. The nurses findings are reviewed. On alternate visits the patient is examined for peripheral vascular disease and foot disease. The doctor checks that the patient is being followed up by an ophthalmic optician or ophthalmologist for diabetic eye disease. If not fundoscopy is performed. An annual audit of results and records is performed. The follow-up interval is between 1 month and 6 months. Approximately 20 patients are seen in each diabetic clinic. The nurse consultation time is approximately 10 minutes. The doctor consultation time is between 10 and 20 minutes.

Advantages – Continuity of care with an annual review. One doctor with a special interest and expertise reviews the patient. The interest is appreciated by the patient as are the shorter waiting times when compared with the diabetic clinic at Poole. The practice has recently acquired the help of a qualified dietitian.

Disadvantages – Other doctors in the practice lose sight of their own diabetic patients. The diabetic clinic tends to be very busy and tends to be something of a 'technical exercise'. Patients see their own family doctors for other problems. The adequacy of hospital follow up has been monitored by the practice diabetic clinic. Those patients lost to follow up by the hospital have been taken over by the practice.

Comment – It will be seen from the above four examples that follow-up can be achieved whether the setting be rural or urban. It is up to the individual family doctors to make a decision as to whether they wish diabetic follow-up to be in the form of a special diabetic clinic within the practice or whether individual partners should see their own patients. However, audit should be undertaken in order to determine whether in fact the follow-up is effective and efficient.

(m) Audit in the Community Care Service

The clinical and biochemical data from all clinics is stored in a DEC-11/23 minicomputer using a Diabetic Data Base (Clinical Data Systems, 41B King Street, Belper, Derbyshire DE5 1PX).

An analysis of these data gives an overview of the service and demographic information to assist in planning. In addition it provides a base for audit in order to assess the quality and to some extent the cost of the service.

13.4 SETTING UP AN INTEGRATED DIABETIC HEALTH CARE SERVICE – A PLAN OF ACTION

The following plan of action is suggested to all those who wish to build a new diabetic service or revise an existing one. The suggestions are based on the experience gained in the formation and development of the Community Care Service for Diabetics in the Poole Area during the 15-year period 1970–1985.

13.4.1 A plan of action

1. A review of district needs.
2. A review of existing diabetic services.
3. Planning the new service.

(a) A review of district needs

Before any real planning can take place it is essential to determine the demography of the district. The population, age, sex and race structure may be obtained from local census. By reviewing population trends during preceding years projected growth patterns may be determined. Knowing the prevalence of diabetes in various age groups and in various races, it is possible to make a good estimate of the number of diabetics requiring care now and in the future. Similarly, knowing the prevalence of diabetic eye disease, it will be possible to make a good estimate of the number of diabetics requiring the attentions of an ophthalmologist. With this background it is possible to review the service as it exists at present and what will be required in the future.

(b) A review of existing diabetic service

A census of the diabetic clinic population should be taken. During the course of a year all patients attending the clinic may be registered on a simple age, sex, race, type of diabetes, family doctor register. This will enable the specialist in charge of the clinic to assess what proportion of the diabetic population he is actually following up. It is likely that in a district without adequate co-operation between primary and secondary health care less than 50% of the patients will be followed up in a diabetic clinic. Many of the patients not followed up in the diabetic clinic will receive a variable standard of care in primary health care with an increased mortality and morbidity (Chapter 6).

The facilities for screening long-term complications of diabetes should be reviewed. Are they adequate? What is happening to those patients who are not followed up in the diabetic clinic?

Is glycaemic control of those patients in the diabetic clinic adequate and what is happening to patients not followed up in the diabetic clinic?

A review of clinics. This must include the number of diabetic clinics operating in the service. Are special provisions made for the review of diabetic eye disease, foot disease and peripheral vascular disease, paediatric patients, obstetric problems, and review clinics?

Table 13.3 shows the time table of the clinics in the Community Care Service for Diabetics in the Poole Area for comparison with other clinics (population served 250 000).

A review of clinic staffing must be made.

Doctors. It has been recommended that one general physician with a special interest in diabetes (i.e. a diabetologist) is required per 100 000 of the population served (Royal College of Physicians of London and British Diabetic Association, 1984).

In addition to specialists, clinics are usually staffed by junior medical staff, and clinical assistants. The use of junior staff in clinics is controversial. There is a conflict between the need to train junior staff and the need for the junior staff to provide a service. Junior staff

Table 13.3 The Community Care Service for diabetics in the Poole area

Clinic	*Day and time*	*No. of patients*	*Staffing*	*Comments*
Diabetic education session	Friday 2–5 p.m. Wednesday 2–5 p.m.	8–12 plus relatives	Diabetic liaison sister, dietitian, chiropodist	Patients to be seen by doctor if indicated. No appointment required.
Meter clinic	Monday	2–3	Diabetic liaison sister	Patients seen as required.
Foot clinic	Friday 2–5 p.m.	Variable	Chiropodists 1 + 1	Foot care film. Patients seen by doctor as required. Runs concurrently with diabetic clinic.
Diabetic review clinic	Monday 1.30–6 p.m.	7–8 new diabetics or diabetics new to the area. 7–8 first return visits.	1 house physician (part of the time) 1 registrar (part of the time) Clinical assistant (2–5 p.m.) Consultant (1.30–6 p.m.)	Diabetic liaison sister in attendance. Education session continues. Transfer to GP. Film shown as required.
Joint retinal clinic (diagnostic & follow-up)	Alternate Tuesdays 9–12	12–16	Consultant ophthalmologist, ophthalmic clinical assistant, diabetologist, research fellow.	Patients from the Poole Community Care Service are filtered by RDH but some direct referrals occur from other parts of the district, e.g. Bournemouth.
Renal clinic (diabetic)	Alternate Tuesdays 9–12	6–10		

Joint retinal clinic (treatment)	Alternate Tuesdays 9–12 R.V. Eye Hosp. Wed. 2–5	3–4 3–4	Consultant ophthalmologist, Ophthalmic clinical assistant	Xenon arc therapy, argon laser.
Medical outpatients	Thursday 2–5.30 p.m.	32–40	Registrar and consultant physician (or other physician)	This is a general medical outpatients but diabetic patients with medical problems are seen in this clinic.
Routine diabetic clinic	Friday 1.30–6 p.m.	50–60	Clinical assistants × 2, registrar × 1, diabetologist × 1 with chiropodists in attendance	The chiropody clinic runs concurrently with this clinic.
Primary health care general practitioner clinics	Monday–Saturday		General practitioners in the area (approximately 150 take part)	Organization left at the discretion of the practices involved.
Primary health care screening programme for diabetic eye disease	Monday–Saturday		Ophthalmic opticians and ophthalmic medical practitioners	2500 patient examinations per annum is the target.

by their very nature are transient and cannot provide good continuity of care. It is probably more efficient and cost effective to employ clinical assistants (e.g. suitable qualified family doctors) on a sessional basis to staff diabetic clinics and provide good continuity of care. Junior staff should work in the clinic supervised by the permanent members of the clinic. They will then receive adequate training and at the same time will be able to do locum work within the clinic to maintain clinic activities during holidays, sickness and study leave. It has been shown that inexperienced junior staff can produce a very inefficient service. In a busy clinic junior staff become anxious and bring patients back to the clinic for follow-up at ever-decreasing intervals. This produces overcrowding within the clinic and more anxiety until eventually the system becomes overburdened and fails.

Nursing staff. It is important to review the function of nurses within diabetic clinics. Qualified and experienced nurses should not be used just as ushers for bringing patients in and out to see the doctor. If their skills are not being utilized then a review of the running of the clinic should be undertaken. Nurses are more than capable for instance of measuring visual acuity, dilating pupils, taking blood pressures, and inspecting feet.

The role of the specialist diabetic nurse was discussed in Chapter 12. It is recommended that a minimum of one specialist diabetic nurse is required per 50 000 of the population served (i.e. per 500 diabetics served).

Dietitian services. Are these adequate, and is the organization efficient?

No staffing norms are available. *Table 13.4* outlines the experience of Poole General Hospital.

Chiropody services. Are these adequate, and are they efficiently organized? It is recommended that two chiropodists per 1000 diabetics – over the age of 65 years are required (see Section 11.6).

Diabetic patient education facilities. What are the existing facilities? Are they adequate, and are they efficient?

Having reviewed the existing diabetic service in the district the question should be asked – is this service satisfactory, and if not can it be improved. The Community Care Service for Diabetics in the

Table 13.4 Dietetic services. No norms are available. Poole General Hospital experience

	Weekly session	
Formal education session	3.0	
New patient follow-up (1:1)	4.5	
Ward patient	6.5	
Domiciliary service	1.0	
Administration and update	1.0	
Total	16.0	sessions
		Each session = 3 hours
i.e. 1.6 dietitians to serve a population of 250 000 (2500 diabetics)		

Based on:
1. Three education sessions/week.
2. Nine new diabetics referred/week.
3. 17 diabetics as inpatients in hospital ward at any time.

Poole Area has shown that 63% of patients can be adequately followed up in primary health care. This is only possible on the basis of a fully shared care system. By sharing the care of the diabetic, clinic facilities are released and may be expanded to improve the service to the patients as a whole.

(c) Planning a new service

Primary health care. If shared care is to be introduced then all patients attending the diabetic clinic should be listed by family doctor. A personal letter should be sent to each family doctor indicating the problems involved in diabetic care with special reference to numbers. A list of his patients attending the diabetic clinic should be enclosed. It should be explained that there would be a controlled transfer to GP care of suitable patients and that audit of outcome would be introduced. The family doctors should be invited to discuss the organizational aspects of shared care at a personal level and at an organized meeting for family doctors. An offer should be made for session/seminars on diabetes in order to improve the background and specialized knowledge of the family doctor. It is essential to stress that a shared care system would be associated with improved facilities for the family doctor and for the diabetic in general.

If ophthalmic opticians are to be asked to co-operate in a Diabetic Eye Disease Screening Programme they should be contacted individually and asked to attend a meeting in order to set up the service (see Chapter 7).

Integration of diabetic care within the hospital should be initiated by joint discussion with paediatricians, obstetricians, geriatricians, surgeons, and ophthalmologists, and all other workers involved in the day-to-day management of the diabetic.

A system of audit should be set up to monitor progress (see Chapter 14).

There should be a planned programme of education for doctors, nurses, and all other staff involved in the shared care service.

No shared care scheme should be undertaken in an area until:

1. There is adequate and proper consultation between hospital and general practitioner.
2. The programme of education is organized for general practitioners, general practice ancillary staff, district nurses and health visitors.
3. A system of communication has been developed.
4. A follow-up and review system can be undertaken in order to monitor the progress of patients both in primary and secondary health care (Hill, 1978).

Secondary health care. Reorganization where necessary of the following services should take place in relation to the needs defined in (a) above.

1. Education sessions.
2. Review clinics.
3. Screening facilities.
4. Special follow-up clinics for long-term complications and problems.
5. The provision of diabetic nurse specialist assistants.
6. Chiropody facilities.
7. Dietetic services.

The specialist should work in close conjunction with the director of laboratory services in order to improve laboratory services to the diabetic and to the family doctor taking part in shared care.

Remember that this cannot be achieved overnight. It represents many years of planning, preparation and development.

(d) The aim: better care

To those who feel that such an undertaking is daunting, perhaps it is worth while remembering the nineteenth century Bishop of Exeter's comment: 'of all work producing results nine tenths must be drudgery.' (Bishop Philpotts)

REFERENCES AND FURTHER READING

Gatling, W., Houston, A.C. and Hill, R.D., (1985) Prevalence of diabetes mellitus in a typical English community. *J. R. Coll. Phys. Lond.*, **19**, 248 (Population statistics.)

Hill, R.D. (1976a) The Community Care Service for Diabetics in the Poole Area. *Br. Med. J.*, **ii**, 1137–39.

Hill, R.D. (1976b) Running a diabetic clinic. *Br. J. Hosp. Med.*, **September**, 218–26.

Hill, R.D. (1978) Shared care for diabetics. *Update*, 1339.

Hill, R.D. (1979) Managing the diabetic patient in general practice. *Mod. Med.*, **July**.

Hill, R.D. (1981) Screening for diabetic retinopathy at the primary health care level. *Diabetologia*, **20**, 670.

Hill, R.D. and Upton, C.E. (1981) Care of the diabetic in the community. *Med. Int.*, **1**, U105–107.

Hill, R.D. (1984) Problems in clinical computing in the diabetic service. *Computer Update*, **January**, 9.

Royal College of Physicians of London (Committee of Endocrinology and Diabetes) and British Diabetic Association (1984) *Report on the Provision of Medical Care for Adult Diabetic Patients in the United Kingdom.*

· Fourteen ·

Audit and planning

14.1 INTRODUCTION

The word audit is derived from the Latine *auditus*. It is variously defined in the Oxford English dictionary as 'a hearing', a searching examination', an examination of accounts', and even 'a day of judgement'. With the coming of Managing Directors to the National Health Service the last definition may become an uncomfortable reality! Audit in diabetes may be regarded as a searching examination.

If time and energy are to be spent on audit the objectives must be clearly defined. These must be:

1. To improve the standard of care.
2. To improve cost-effectiveness.

The objectives therefore define what we are to measure in order to carry out a searching examination. If planning is to be effective it must be based on hard data. Trends observed over a period of time must be taken into account when planning and developing the system.

The minimum data set required for patient identification, communication, and demographic data is as follows:

1. Patient identification:
   (i) Surname.
   (ii) Forename (s).
   (iii) Title.
   (iv) NHS number
   (v) Hospital number.
2. Communications:
   (i) Patient address.
   (ii) Patient telephone number.
   (iii) GP name.

(iv) GP address.
(v) GP telephone number.
(vi) GP FPC Number.
(vii) Hospital consultant name.
(viii) Other name.
(ix) Other address.

3. Demographic data.
   (i) Date of birth.
   (ii) Sex.
   (iii) Race.
   (iv) Date of diagnosis.
   (v) Treatment group NIDD diet, NIDD OHA, NIDD I, and IDD.
   (vi) Smoking habits.
   (vii) Social class.

It defines the patient as a unique individual within the service, and provides data required for essential communication.

If care and cost comparisons are to be made either within a given diabetic service or between different services in different parts of the country, it is essential to be certain that the standard of care achieved and the costs involved are being compared in similar populations. It is therefore vital to collect demographic data. The minimum data set defines the necessary demographic data. By observing the changing pattern of demographic data planning information will be obtained.

14.2 AUDIT OF CARE

If audit is to mean anything there must be some standardization of care performance indicators. These may be grouped as follows:

1. Glycaemic control:
   (i) Blood glucose (IBS, FBS, PP, RBS).
   (ii) HbA1 (? percentage above upper limit of normal).
   (iii) Lipids.
2. Routine follow-up:
   (i) Place of follow-up (Diabetic Clinic/GP/Nil).
   (ii) Frequency of follow-up (date of follow-up).
   (ii) Height/Weight/BMI).

3. Long-term complications:
   (i) Eyes:
   Place of eye follow-up.
   Frequency of eye follow-up (date of follow-up).
   Distant visual acuity right and left.
   Cataract.
   Retinopathy – classify.
   (ii) Kidneys:
   Microalbuminuria (albumin/creatinine ratio and albumin excretion rate).
   Persistent albuminuria.
   Serum creatinine.
   (iii) Peripheral vascular disease:
   Intermittent claudication (claudicating distance).
   Ischaemic skin.
   Ischaemic ulceration.
   Large vessel surgery.
   Amputation (levels).
   (iv) Nerves:
   Subjective peripheral neuropathy.
   Objective neuropathy.
   Vibration threshold.
   Autonomic neuropathy (classify).
   (v) Coronary artery disease:
   ECG changes only.
   Angina pectoris.
   Myocardial infarction.
   Coronary artery bypass surgery.
   (vi) Cerebrovascular disease:
   Transient ischaemic attack.
   Stroke.
   (vii) Hypertension:
   Blood pressure.
   Treatment.
4. Morbidity and mortality:
   (i) Admission data – date of admission, date of discharge, diagnosis.
   (ii) Date of death, cause of death, PM, no PM.

The collection of the above data will enable the diabetic service to assess:

1. The standard of control achieved.
2. The frequency of follow-up.
3. Prevalence and incidence of long-term complications.
4. The mortality and morbidity within the service.

This will enable thought provoking comparisons to be made within the service, and, taking into account demographic data, comparisons with other services.

14.2.1 Audit of education

A prominent feature of the modern diabetic service is the educational program. It is essential to audit what is being achieved in terms of what is learnt by the patients. This does not necessarily mean an alteration in behaviour on the part of the patient but by linking the educational assessment with the standards of control achieved an assessment of compliance can be made. The areas that might be used in the assessment of knowledge gained by patient when attending the diabetic education session are as follows:

1. What is diabetes?
2. What is a diabetic diet?
3. Glycaemic control.
4. Home monitoring – urine/blood tests.
5. Oral hypoglycaemic agents.
6. Insulin therapy – storage, injection, dose adjustment.
7. Hyperglycaemia and illness.
8. Hypoglycaemia.
9. Driving.

Each of the above areas should be related to a norm for the clinic before and after the educational programme. An assessment of compliance should be included. Computer assisted learning programmes are now available with associated computerized assessment. This will enable the educator to audit the educational programme and to assess its effectiveness in terms of information gained by the patient (Wise, P. also Ames Diabetes Management System).

14.3 USING AUDIT OF CARE

The collection of the data outlined above should enable us to answer the following questions:

1. What is the population at risk and how is it changing?
2. Who is providing the care?
3. Is our diabetic education service effective?
4. Is our follow-up effective?
5. What are the standards of glycaemic control being achieved?
6. Is screening for long-term complications effective?
7. Are we affecting morbidity and mortality?

14.3.1 Health care planning

Demographic data provides important information for use in health care planning. In 1971 an investigation into population growth and its projections into the future revealed a somewhat frightening situation in Poole. *Table 13.1* demonstrates the rise in population. It was this rise in the population which prompted the formation of the Community Care Service for Diabetics in the Poole Area. Without this the Diabetic Service would now have been overwhelmed by numbers (Hill, 1976).

14.3.2 Assessment of care

Audit will also provide an insight into diabetes management practices within a health care district. *Table 14.1* shows methods of treatment in two sample populations.

In the Poole sample, 60% of the patients have diabetes treated with diet, or a diet together with an oral hypoglycaemic agent; 40% of

Table 14.1 Methods of treatment

	Poole	*London*
Population sample	2315	217
Diet ± OHA	60%	80%
Insulin	40%	20%

OHA = Oral hypoglycaemic agent.

patients are treated with insulin (Gatling, W., MD thesis). This makes an interesting comparison with the figures of Yudkin in his Tower Hamlets survey from London (Yudkin *et al.*, 1980). In this survey only 20% of patients were being treated with insulin. These figures, however, must be related to the demographic structure of the population and should also be related to the standards of control achieved. At the very least they should prompt thoughts as to why discrepancies of this nature exist.

To assess the efficiency and effectiveness of the service being provided the place of follow-up must be known. It should be possible to calculate the frequency of follow-up from the record. Similarly, the standard of glycaemic control may be assessed in terms of blood glucose and haemoglobin A1 values. However, there are problems here. The blood glucose may be fasting (FBS), 2 hours post prandial (IBS), preprandial (PP) or random (RBS). The methods of measuring blood glucose and HbA1 are numerous and norms must be established.

Table 14.2 shows a comparison between the glycaemic control obtained in Poole (Gatling, W., MD thesis) and Tower Hamlets in London (Yudkin *et al.*, 1980).

The first important difference to be noted is that in Poole 63% of the patients are provided with diabetic care in general practice compared with 54% in London. This might be expected because of the shared care scheme operating in Poole (Hill, 1976). No figures for interval blood sugar are available from London but the comparison between patients managed in Poole general practice with those of the hospital is interesting. The comparison is a reasonable one in

Table 14.2 Glycaemic control in two districts

	%	*IBS*	*HbA1*
Gatling (Poole, 1985)			
Hospital	37	9.6*	9.3*
GP	63	8.9*	8.8**
Yudkin (London, 1980)			
Hospital	46	—	13.4
GP	54	—	13.2

* P <0.01; ** P <0.001.

that the blood glucose levels are measured 2 hours after a meal (interval blood sugar) both for general practice and hospital. The blood glucose is measured in the same laboratory by the same method for the two groups. It will be seen that the standard of control achieved by the family doctors is better than that achieved by the hospital ($P < 0.01$). There is a marked difference between HbA1 values measured in Poole and those measured in London. This is due mainly to the difference in methodology. However, comparing GP group with hospital group it will be seen that in Poole again the GPs achieve a better standard of control ($P < 0.001$) and in London there is no difference between the groups. To interpret these results it is important to know demographic details. Examination of the two populations shows that they are different and no direct comparison can be made. In addition to this in Poole we would expect the patients in general practice to be better controlled than those looked after in hospital since it is our policy to transfer to GP care those patients who are well controlled and have no complications.

Tables 14.3 and *14.4* show the problems of demography, terminology and methodology when making comparisons between centres. Here we not only have the problem of populations of different structure being compared but also the problem of terminology. It is impossible to group the patients in terms of treatment. Insulin-dependent diabetics are not distinguished clearly from non-insulin dependent diabetics taking insulin in order to achieve better control.

In each of the centres listed HbA1 is measured by a different method. One way of overcoming this is to express the value as a percentage of the upper limit of normal (% ULN).

By collecting information on the presence of long-term complications it is possible to establish the prevalence and incidence of diabetic eye disease, peripheral vascular disease, neuropathy, nephropathy and foot disease. By recording the frequency of follow-up it will be possible to assess the efficiency of a service in terms of facilities or early detection and treatment.

In order to assess the data collected comparison will be made with established norms, between one diabetic service and another, between groups of patients within a given service and between groups of patients with the mean for the whole service.

From the above it will be seen that careful standardization of data is absolutely essential if any meaningful comparisons and assessments are to be made.

Table 14.3 Standard of control—blood glucose (mmol/l)

	Leeds (1984)★	*Poole (1985)*†
All diabetics	9.8	9.1
Insulin taking	10.45	9.5
Not taking insulin	9.25	9.0

★ Stickland *et al.* (1984).
† Gatling, W. (1985).

Table 14.4 Standard of control — HbA1 (%)

	Leeds (1984)★	*London (1980)*†	*Poole (1985)*‡
All diabetics	10.05 (134%)	13.1 (125%)	9.0 (113%)
Insulin taking	10.5 (140%)	14.88 (142%)	9.5 (119%)
Not taking insulin	9.55 (127%)	12.84 (122%)	8.8 (110%)
ULN	7.5	10.5	8.0

ULN = upper limit normal (%ULN).
★ Stickland *et al.* (1984).
† Yudkin *et al.* (1980).
‡ Gatling, W. (1985).

14.4 AUDIT OF COSTS

The cost of diabetic care forms a small but significant part of the cost of the overall expenses incurred in primary and secondary health care. It would be impossible to undertake absolute costing for such activities as follow-up consultation, education, dietetics, chiropody, screening for long-term complications, admissions, pharmaceuticals and consumables, and staffing. It would probably be very difficult and unrewarding to cost each item in terms of rent and lighting, for instance. Here again we should opt for a minimum data set in order to cost the care we are providing. It is probably worth while costing the most expensive items. These are undoubtedly pharmaceuticals, consumables, staff, and the cost of admissions:

1. Yearly expenditure on pharmaceuticals:
   (i) Insulin
   (ii) Oral hypoglycaemic agents
   (ii) Other
2. Yearly expenditure on consumables:
   (i) Syringes.
   (ii) Needles.
   (iii) Blood testing.
   (iv) Urine testing.
3. Yearly expenditure on staff.
4. Yearly expenditure on admissions.

Many pharmacie are now equipped with computing systems (e.g. 'Horis') which collect the necessary data and make audit possible. A head count of staff involved in diabetic care is also possible and a reasonable costing can be made. Similarly, the cost of admissions can be calculated.

14.5 USING AUDIT OF COSTS

Armed with this type of information it becomes possible to undertake cost cutting exercises. As an example it is worth while looking at insulin delivery systems. In 1982 our expenditure on glass insulin syringes was £3210. With the coming of U-100 insulin patients were advised to use plastic syringes and at a cost of 10p per week were advised to purchase their own. The syringe bill dropped to £260 per annum. It is likely that in 1985 the cost will be significantly less.

Similarly a comparison may be made between an insulin 'starter

Table 14.5 Insulin 'starter pack' — cost in £

1982	
Two glass syringes	10.00
Needles (reusable)	5.00
Industrial spirit	70
Carrying case	1.76
Cotton wool	70
Total	18.16
1984	
20 U-100 disposable syringes	1.60

Table 14.6 Cost of blood test strip

	Poole	*St. Elsewhere*
Population	230 000	200 000
Age 65 or over	17%	34%
Strips:cost p.a.	£3200	£5300

pack' in 1982 and that given in 1984. *Table 14.5* shows the comparable costs. It will be seen that the change in policy from glass syringes to disposable syringes has once again produced a saving.

Considerable savings are also possible by monitoring the costs of insulin. By negotiating prices with companies and bulk buying it has been possible to reduce the cost of insulin by £1 per vial. This is a saving of 16% and on our twice daily regimen represents a saving of £1500 per annum alone.

With the coming of home blood glucose monitoring a considerable cost is now involved in the provision of blood test strips. *Table 14.6* shows a cost comparison between Poole and St. Elsewhere.

It will be seen that the population of Poole is slightly greater and the age structure such that one would expect more insulin-treated diabetics to be present in the population. Despite this the expenditure on blood testing strips by Poole is only £3200 per annum compared with £5300 per annum. This should give pause for thought. Are we in Poole perhaps undermonitoring blood glucose in the population? Of course, it could be that St. Elsewhere is overmonitoring blood glucose in the population. Whichever is the answer this information should stimulate a searching examination of the reasons for this discrepancy.

From what has been written it may be seen that audit in diabetes is not only possible but worth while. It must contain an index of performance related both to population and costs. Costs must be related both to population and to performance. If this type of effort is to provide useful information it is essential that minimum data sets of performance indicators and costs be clearly defined and standardized.

14.6 CONCLUSION – WHAT WE NEED TO DO

1. Decide to audit or not to audit.
2. Standardize a minimum data set – performance indicators.

3. Standardize a minimum data set – costs.
4. Collect the data of the minimum data sets and store in a suitable computer (Hill, 1986).
5. Provide software programmes to analyse the data in a standard form to allow useful comparisons.

REFERENCES

The Ames Diabetes Management System Computer comprises:

- Computer
- Printer
- Software Package

Obtainable as a package deal: Ames Division, Miles Laboratories Ltd., PO Box 27, Stoke Court, Stoke Poges, Slough, SL2 4LY, England.

Gatling, W. (1986) *The Prevalence of Diabetic Nephropahy*, DM Thesis, Southampton University.

Gatling, W., Houston, A.C. and Hill, R.D. (1985) The prevalence of diabetes mellitus in a typical English community. *J. R. Coll. Phys. Lond.*, **19**, 248–50.

Hill, R.D. (1976) The Community Care Service for Diabetics in the Poole Area. *Br. Med. J.*, **ii**, 1137–39.

Hill, R.D. (1986) Report of the B.D.A. Working Party on Computing in Diabetes. *Practical Diabetes* (as a series).

Stickland, M.H. *et al.* (1984) Haemoglobin A1C concentrations in men and women with diabetes. *Br. Med. J.*, **289**, 733.

Wise, P. *Micro Base System for Learning and Assessment.* Details from Dr Peter Wise, Consultant Physician, Charing Cross Hospital (Fulham), Fulham Palace Road, London W6 8RF.

Yudkin, J.S. Boucher, B.J., Schopflin, K.E. *et al.* (1980) The quality of diabetic care in a London health district. *J. Epidemiol. Commun. Hlth.*, **34**, 277–80.

· Appendix one ·

Demography

A1.1 INTRODUCTION

Demography describes the structure of a population in statistical terms. Knowing the demographic details of a population and the prevalence of any condition, the total number of patients expected to have that condition may be calculated. However, if the population under consideration is not homogeneous, errors creep in. The more heterogeneous the population the greater the error. The more accurate demographic statistics in relation to age, sex and racial structure, the more accurate will estimates be.

Accurate population statistics collected over the years will give an indication of rates of change in that population and allow service requirements to be estimated for the future. Detailed information provides ammunition in the battle for the allocation of resources. It enables a logical assessment of the service as it stands at present, and planning for the service requirements of the future.

A1.2 WHAT YOU NEED TO KNOW

For large populations demographic data may be obtained from local census reports. This will give information on the total number served, together with the age, sex and sometimes racial structure of the population. In the family doctor practice the construction of an age/sex register will provide important information on the structure of the population served.

Remember, the more detailed the demographic data the more accurate the estimate you can make. However, even the rough estimate of the total population you serve will enable a rough estimate of the number of patients with diabetes which you might expect to have under your care.

The total number of diabetics in the population which you serve may be calculated from the crude prevalence (in the UK, 1.01%). However, this is only a rough estimation for a population having 'the typical age/sex/racial structure of the UK' (Gatling, 1986).

For a more accurate assessment it is essential to take note of the effect of the age and sex structure of the population. *Tables A.1–A1.3* below indicate the age/sex structure of the UK. The prevalence of diabetes for each age group is shown in *Tables A1.4–A1.6*. It will be seen that the effect of age is profound. Therefore when calculating the number of diabetics within the community you serve you must know the proportions in the different age groups before an accurate figure can be obtained.

Table A1.1 Age distribution of all the patients registered with the 40 GPs in the study and comparison with UK (Gatling, 1986)

Age in years	*No. of patients registered*	%	*% UK*
Under 5	5497	6.1	6.1
5–14	12 176	13.4	14.7
15–29	17 961	19.8	22.5
30–44	19 309	21.3	19.5
45–64	20 214	22.3	22.3
65–74	9204	10.2	9.2
75 and over	6207	6.8	5.7
Unknown	92	0.1	
Total	90 660	100	100

1981 Census figures. Office of Population Censuses and Surveys.

Table A1.2 Age distribution of the male patients registered with the 40 GPs in the study and comparison with UK (Gatling, 1986)

Age in years	*No. of patients registered*	%	*UK (%)*
Under 5	2836	6.5	6.4
5–14	6482	14.9	15.5
15–29	8762	20.2	23.5
30–44	9336	21.5	20.2
45–64	9740	22.4	22.4
65–74	4035	9.3	8.2
75 and over	2234	5.1	3.8
Unknown	45	0.1	
Total	43 470	100	100

1981 Census figures. Office of Population Censuses and Surveys.

Table A1.3 Age distribution of the female patients registered with the 40 GPs in the study and comparison with UK (Gatling, 1986)

Age in years	*No. of patients registered*	%	*UK (%)*
Under 5	2661	5.6	5.8
5–14	5694	12.1	13.9
15–29	9199	19.5	21.6
30–44	9973	21.1	19.0
45–64	10 474	22.2	22.3
65–74	5169	11.0	10.0
75 and over	3973	8.4	7.4
Unknown	47	0.1	
Total	47 190	100	100

1981 Census figures. Office of Population Censuses and Surveys.

Table A1.4 Age-specific rate for diabetes mellitus in the study population (Gatling, 1986)

Age in years	*No. of patients registered*	*No. of diabetics*	*Rate per 1000*
Under 5	5497	0	<0.18
5–14	12 176	16	1.3
15–29	17 961	70	4.0
30–44	19 309	93	4.8
45–64	20 214	259	12.8
65–74	9204	262	28.5
75 and over	6207	217	35.0
Unknown	92		
Total	90 660	917	

Table A1.5 Age-specific rate of diabetes mellitus in the male population (Gatling, 1986)

Age in years	*No. of patients registered*	*No. of diabetics*	*Rate per 1000*
Under 5	2836	0	<0.18
5–14	6482	10	1.5
15–29	8762	36	4.1
30–44	9336	43	4.6
45–64	9740	154	15.8
65–74	4035	134	33.2
75 and over	2234	102	45.7
Unknown	45		
Total	43 470	479	

Table A1.6 Age-specific rate for diabetes mellitus in the female population (Gatling, 1986)

Age in years	*No. of patients registered*	*No. of diabetics*	*Rate per 1000 female study population*
Under 5	2661	0	<0.18
5–14	5694	6	1.1
15–29	9199	34	3.7
30–44	9973	50	5.0
45–64	10 474	105	10.0
65–74	5169	128	24.8
75 and over	3973	115	29.0
Unknown	47		
Total	47 190	438	

The number of insulin dependent and non-insulin dependent diabetics may be calculated from *Table A1.7*.

Table A1.7 Proportion of categories of diabetes within the community (Adapted from Gatling, 1986)

Treatment	*% all*	*% NIDD*
Diet only	20.1	26.4
Oral hypoglycaemic agent	40.4	53.1
Insulin	39.5	20.5

NIDD = non-insulin dependent diabetics.

A1.3 THE EFFECT OF RACE

An accurate picture of the racial structure of the population served may not be readily available and yet it may have a profound effect on the prevalence of diabetes and its complications. The situation is complicated by the fact that people who have settled in other parts of the world do not have the same prevalence of diabetes as similar populations in their homeland. People from the Indian sub continent seem to be particularly susceptible to diabetes. Thus although the prevalence of diabetes in India is not so very different to that in the UK, the prevalence of diabetes in an age-adjusted community of people living in the UK originating from India is at least 3.8 times higher than for the European population. Here again the age group must be taken into consideration. For the age group 40–64 years the prevalence is five times that of a similar European population. In the 50–59 year age group it reaches no less than 8% and in the 60–69 year group it reaches 12%.

There are more than one million Asians in the UK and clearly they must be taken into account when planning services for a population containing any substantial minority group.

For details on other racial groups the reader is referred to the list of references and further reading.

A1.4 THE LONG-TERM COMPLICATIONS OF DIABETES

Knowing the number of diabetics served it is possible to estimate the number of patients with retinopathy (see Chapter 7) and nephropathy (*Table A1.8*).

Table A1.8 Diabetic renal disease (adapted from Gatling, 1986)

Chronic renal failure (serum creatinine greater than 150 μmol/l)	3.8%
At risk raised RA/C ratio	38%
raised AER	30%

RA = Urinary albumin concentration (μg/100 ml); C = urinary creatinine concentration (μmol/l) in random sample or urine.
AER = Albumin excretion rate.

A1.5 CONCLUSION

Demographic and prevalence data are important in planning for the care of diabetic patients and for evaluating existing services. The specialist in diabetic care must know his population, evaluate his own service, and plan for the future.

REFERENCES AND FURTHER READING

Gatling, W. (1986) *The Prevalence of Diabetic Nephropathy*, DM, University of Southampton.

R.J. Jarrett, (1986) *Diabetes Mellitus. Series in Clinical Epidemiology*, Croom Helm, London.

Mann, J.I., Pyorala, K. and Teuscher, A. (1983) *Diabetes in Epidemiological Perspective*, Churchill Livingstone, London.

Mather, H.M. and Keen, H. (1985) The Southall Diabetes Survey: prevalence of known diabetes in Asians and Europeans. *Br. Med. J.*, **291**, 1081–4.

· Appendix two ·

Home/self blood glucose monitoring (H/S BGM)

The maintenance of normal or near-normal glycaemia is now accepted as a major goal in the management of patients with diabetes mellitus. By so doing it is hoped to reduce the incidence of, or at the very least delay the onset of long-term complications. The maintenance of normal or near-normal glycaemia in pregnancy is mandatory. The advantages are clear cut and well documented.

In diabetes mellitus blood glucose concentration fluctuates widely throughout the day and night. This is particularly so in insulin-dependent diabetics. It is therefore clear that a single isolated blood glucose estimation when a patient attends the clinic is inadequate in assessing the standard of control achieved. It is clearly of little use when attempting to advise the patient on changes in treatment to improve the standard of control. The haemoglobin A1 estimation now gives a better indication of overall glycaemia control but does not help in the daily adjustment of treatment.

Urine testing as a means of monitoring the standard of glycaemic control achieved has long been known to be inadequate. At best it is semi-quantitative and does not accurately reflect the concomitant blood glucose value. This may be due to the rapidly changing blood glucose values during the collection of urine in the bladder and the variability of the renal threshold for glucose. In the past urine tests were the only available method for monitoring the standard of control achieved but now more sophisticated blood glucose methods are available.

The information provided by blood glucose testing in the home provides information on the standard of control achieved over long periods of time and in addition to this gives feedback information allowing the patient to adjust treatment and improve self-care.

A2.1 ADVANTAGES OF HOME/SELF BLOOD GLUCOSE MONITORING

1. Blood glucose may be determined at any time of the day or night.
2. A true picture of the blood glucose level and variability is obtained in the home/work environment.
3. Instant feedback is given to the patient allowing adjustment of treatment.

A2.2 DISADVANTAGES OF HOME/SELF BLOOD GLUCOSE MONITORING

1. Blood glucose monitoring intrudes into every-day life adding yet another burden to the existing problem of medication/insulin injection/diet. However, despite this most patients prefer blood glucose monitoring and find it more acceptable than urine testing.
2. The method is invasive and requireds a finger prick which may be painful.
3. Test strips and meters are expensive.

A2.3 WHO SHOULD CARRY OUT HOME/SELF BLOOD GLUCOSE MONITORING?

A2.3.1 Absolute indications

1. During pregnancy
2. Known insulin-treated diabetics with haemoglobin A1 values greater than normal and/or hypoglcaemia.
3. Newly diagnosed insulin-treated diabetics from diagnosis even when blood glucose and HbA1 values are within the normal range. By doing this confidence is instilled into the patient and the habit of home blood glucose monitoring with adjustments of insulin is established from the onset.

A2.3.2 Relative indication

Any patient, either insulin treated or non-insulin treated with poor control or suspected hypoglycaemia.

A2.4 GLUCOSE TESTING STRIPS AVAILABLE

1. Dextrostix (Ames).
2. Visidex II (Ames).
3. Glucostix (Ames).
4. BM Glycemie Test Strips (known in different countries by different names):
   (i) Chamstrip BG (USA and Canada).
   (ii) BM Test Glycemie 20–800R/1–44 (Australia and New Zealand).
   (iii) Haemo-Gluko Test 20–800 (all countries in Europe except UK).
   (iv) BM Test Glycemie 1–44 (UK).

A2.5 OBTAINING A SPECIMEN OF BLOOD

The object is to produce sufficient blood by finger prick to cover the reagent pad on the test strip. The instructions given by the manufacturer must be followed if accurate readings are to be obtained.

The edges of the fingers should be pricked. It is important not to prick the sensitive pulp area of the fingers. This is painful and tends to inhibit testing. The ear lobe may sometimes be used. It is not necessary to swab the finger before pricking. Indeed, substances used for swabbing fingers may in fact damage the sensitive enzymes in the reagent pads. Warm hands assist the production of sufficient quantities of blood and patients should be advised to wash their hands in warm soapy water before performing the test.

A suitable lancet should be used to prick the finger. Hypodermic needles should not be used as these give a small deep puncture which is painful and produces little blood. Some patients prefer to use machines that automatically prick the finger and help the faint hearted (e.g. GLUCOLET (Ames), but many other devices are on the market). The drop of blood obtained should be placed on to the reagent pad of the test strip making sure that the whole pad is covered with blood. The blood should be left in contact with the pad according to the manufacturer's instructions. The time varies from make to make. After the prescribed period the blood should be washed off (Dextrostix) or wiped off (other test strips). The glucose in the blood interacts with reagents on the test strip to generate a colour. The amount of colour developed depends on the amount of glucose in the blood. Depending on the test used, the blood sugar level may be determined either by visually comparing the colour of the test strip against a colour scale provided or by using a meter. It is essential to use a meter specifically designed to read the test strip used.

A2.6 METERS

Some patients have no difficulty in comparing the colour generated on the test strip with the colour scale provided on the strip container. However, many patients prefer to use a meter to read the strip. The author prefers patients to use a meter and in clinical practice has found this to be the most useful in teaching the patient to adjust his or her own insulin dosage. On the other hand, it must be stated that meters are expensive and that some investigators have found little advantage in their use. In addition to this there may be a false sense of security for the patient in believing that the meter is always right.

Many different meters have been produced to read the various test strips available. Some examples are given below:

1. The Glucometer (Ames) will read glucose values between 1 and 22 mmol/1 using Dextrostix (Plate 24).
2. The Glucometer II (Ames) will read blood glucose values 2–22 mmol/1 using Glucostix.
3. The Reflolux II, Reflolux, will read BM Test Glycaemi 1–44 (BCL, Bochringer Mannheim).
4. Hypocount (Hypoguard Limited).
5. Glucocheck SC (Medistron).

When performed properly, self-monitoring is not only accurate but is reliable and effective. It provides an effective tool for teaching the diabetic how every-day life affects blood glucose levels and how these may be controlled by adjusting food intake, exercise, and insulin dose. It is also helpful in detecting hypoglycaemia. The knowledge that the patient is in command has a positive psychological impact and improves the patient's confidence. The possible reduction in frequency of follow-up and laboratory visits also makes home/self blood glucose monitoring cost effective.

Recently, meters have been produced which contain a memory chip, e.g. Glucometer – M (Ames). Such meters automatically store information on date, time, blood glucose, and events. This information may be retrieved in the clinic using simple equipment and a printout provided for the notes. This again provides an excellent educational tool for teaching patients how to adjust the insulin and obtain good glycaemic control.

A2.7 SOURCES OF ERROR

In the presence of conflicting results between haemoglobin A1 values, laboratory blood glucose values, and home/self blood glucose monitoring, it is important to look for possible sources of error. These are listed below:

1. Insufficient blood to cover reagent pad.
2. Inaccurate timing.
3. Incorrect washing, blotting or wiping blood off the test strip.
4. Dirty optical systems in the meter.
5. Lack of calibration of meter.
6. Deliberate falsification of results.

· Appendix three ·

Continuous subcutaneous insulin infusion (CSII)

A3.1 INTRODUCTION

Continuous subcutaneous insulin infustion using small portable pumps may be used in selected patients to achieve improved glycaemic control. Such a course of action should not be undertaken lightly. It requires a considerable commitment from both patient and diabetic team.

A3.2 INDICATIONS

A3.2.1 Absolute indications

There are no absolute indications for CSII.

A3.2.2 Relative indications

1. Painful neuropathy.
2. Labile diabetes, particularly with recurrent hypoglycaemia.
3. Irregular life style where flexibility is paramount.
4. Poor glycaemic control during pregnancy despite multiple injections of insulin.

A3.3 CONTRAINDICATIONS

A3.3.1 Absolute contraindictions

1. Failure of the patient to accept basic and special education.
2. Failure of the patient to accept the necessity for frequent and regular self blood glucose monitoring.
3. An inability of the diabetic team to provide the patient with the necessary education.

4. Inability of the diabetic team to provide the patient with adequate supervision and training.
5. Failure of the diabetic team to provide a 24 hour on-call service (phone/clinic/ward).
6. Recurrent skin infection.

A3.3.2 Relative contraindictions

1. Brittle diabetes.
2. Severe autonomic neuropathy.
3. Chronic renal failure.

A3.4 DANGERS AND PROBLEMS OF CSII

1. Rapid metabolic decompensation leading to diabetic keto-acidosis.
2. Recurrent infections at the site of the infusion.
3. The danger of deterioration of retinopathy.
4. Costs.
5. Increased workload for diabetic service staff.

A3.4.1 CSII – Which pump?

Table A3.1 gives details of ten pumps (Sleigholm *et al.*, 1986)

Note: *Table A.3.1* shows the cost of purchase in sterling (without VAT) as at 1/4/85, as well as the annual running costs. The cost of insulin is not included in this estimate, except for the Nordisk Infuser, which uses cartridges of Velosulin, which are priced at a premium of approximately 20% compared with standard vials. A patient using normal vials of insulin would consume an average of 20× 10 ml vials per annum, at a cost of approximately £148 inc VAT.

REFERENCES

Sleightholm, M.A., Roberts, M. and Kohner, E.M. (1986) 'Which pump'? *Practical Diabetes*, **3**, 238.

Ward, J., (1986) Guidelines for using insulin infusion pumps. *Update Diabetes*, **9**, 1.

Table A3.1 Details of ten pumps

Pump	*Size* (cm)	*Weight* (g)	*Cost* £	*Running cost* (£)	*Technical rating*	*Patient rating*
Mill Hill 1000	14×7.3×3.5	308	*	106	10	6
Mill Hill 1001	15×7.3×2.5	288	*	106	9	7
Graseby MS-26	16×7.3×2.5	190	*	98	8	8
Autosyringe AS-6M	16×8.6×2.5	272	674	190	5	—
Autosyringe AS-6MP	16×8.6×2.5	272	950	190	4	2
Betatron I	9.9×6.6×2	163	1300	236	3	—
Betatron II	9.9×6.6×2	163	1500	236	1	1
Ames Microjet	17×7×2	300	650	214	7	4
Nordisk Infuser	10×6×2	188	750	345†	6	5
Graseby MS-36	12×6×2.5	133	495	88	2	3

* Not in production.
† Includes extra cost of insulin cartridges.

· Appendix four ·

Desirable weights

Table A4.1 Desirable weights for men over the age of 25 years, calculated according to frame size allowing for indoor clothing. Male heights allow for 1″ heels. Derived from Metropolitan Life Insurance Company Data.

Height		*Small frame*		*Medium frame*		*Large frame*	
Ft/in	cm	Stone/lb	kg	Stone/lb	kg	Stone/lb	kg
5.2	157.5	8.0–8.8	50.8–54.4	8.6–9.3	53.5–58.5	9.0–10.1	57.2–64.0
5.3	160.0	8.3–8.11	52.2–55.8	8.9–9.7	54.9–60.3	9.3–10.4	58.5–65.3
5.4	162.6	8.6–9.0	53.5–57.2	8.12–9.10	56.2–61.7	9.6–10.8	59.9–67.1
5.5	165.1	8.9–9.3	54.9–58.5	9.1–9.13	57.6–63.0	9.9–10.12	61.2–68.9
5.6	167.6	8.12–9.7	56.2–60.3	9.4–10.3	59.0–64.9	9.12–11.2	62.6–70.8
5.7	170.2	9.2–9.11	58.1–62.1	9.8–10.7	60.8–66.7	10.2–11.7	64.4–73.0
5.8	172.7	9.6–10.1	59.9–64.0	9.12–10.12	62.6–68.9	10.7–11.12	66.7–75.3
5.9	175.3	9.10–10.5	61.7–65.8	10.2–11.2	64.4–70.8	10.11–12.2	68.5–77.1
5.10	177.8	10.0–10.10	63.5–68.0	10.6–11.6	66.2–72.6	11.1–12.6	70.3–78.9
5.11	180.3	10.4–11.0	65.3–69.9	10.10–11.11	68.0–74.8	11.5–12.11	72.1–81.2
6.0	182.9	10.8–11.4	67.1–71.7	11.0–12.2	69.9–77.1	11.10–13.2	74.3–83.5
6.1	185.4	10.12–11.8	68.9–73.5	11.4–12.7	71.7–79.4	12.0–13.7	76.2–85.7
6.2	188.0	11.2–11.13	70.8–75.8	11.8–12.12	73.5–81.6	12.5–13.12	78.5–88.0
6.3	190.5	11.6–12.3	72.6–77.6	11.13–13.3	75.8–83.9	12.10–14.3	80.7–90.3
6.4	193.0	11.10–12.7	74.4–79.4	12.4–13.8	78.0–86.2	13.0–14.8	86.2–92.5

Table A4.2 Desirable weights for women over the age of 25 years, calculated according to frame size allowing for indoor clothing. Female heights allow for 2″ heels. Derived from Metropolitan Life Insurance Company Data

Height		*Small frame*		*Medium frame*		*Large frame*	
Ft/in	cm	Stone/lb	kg	Stone/lb	kg	Stone/lb	kg
4.10	147.3	6.8–7.0	41.7–44.5	6.12–7.9	43.5–48.5	7.6–8.7	47.2–54.0
4.11	149.9	6.10–7.3	42.6–45.8	7.0–7.12	44.5–50.0	7.8–8.10	48.1–55.3
5.0	152.4	6.12–7.6	43.5–47.2	7.3–8.1	45.8–51.3	7.11–8.13	49.4–56.7
5.1	154.9	7.1–7.9	44.9–48.5	7.6–8.4	47.2–52.6	8.0–9.2	50.8–58.1
5.2	157.5	7.4–7.12	46.3–50.0	7.9–8.7	48.5–54.0	8.3–9.5	52.2–59.4
5.3	160.0	7.7–8.1	47.6–51.3	7.12–8.10	50.0–55.3	8.6–9.12	54.9–62.6
5.4	162.6	7.10–8.4	49.0–52.6	8.0–9.0	50.8–57.2	8.6–9.8	53.5–60.8
5.5	165.1	7.13–8.87	50.3–54.0	8.4–9.4	52.6–59.0	8.13–10.2	56.7–64.4
5.6	167.6	8.2–8.11	51.7–55.8	8.8–9.9	54.4–61.2	9.3–10.6	58.5–66.2
5.7	170.2	8.6–9.1	53.5–57.6	8.12–9.13	56.2–63.0	9.7–10.10	60.3–68.0
5.8	172.7	8.10–9.5	55.3–59.4	9.2–10.3	58.1–64.9	9.11–11.0	62.1–69.9
5.9	175.3	9.0–9.9	57.2–61.2	9.6–10.7	59.9–66.7	10.1–11.4	64.0–71.7
5.10	177.8	9.4–10.0	59.0–63.5	9.10–10.11	61.0–68.5	10.5–11.9	65.8–73.9
5.11	180.3	9.8–10.4	60.8–65.3	10.0–11.1	63.5–70.3	10.9–12.0	67.6–76.2
6.0	182.9	9.12–10.8	62.6–67.1	10.4–11.5	65.3–72.1	10.13–12.5	69.4–78.5

Glossary

A

Acidaemia	An excess of acid in the blood.
Afferent arteriole	The smallest branch of the renal artery supplying blood to the glomerulus.
Albumin	A protein in the blood.
Amaurosis fugax	Transient recurrent loss of vision.
Amyotrophy	Muscular wasting.
Angina pectoris	Chest pain due to coronary artery disease
Angiography	A means of outlining the blood vessels using X-rays after the injection of a radio-opaque substance.
Angioplasty	Opening up the lumen of narrowed blood vessels.
Anuria	The cessation of the production of urine.
Asteriod hyalosis (hyalitis)	Asteroid, star-like; hyalosis (hyalitis) referring to the clear glass-like vitreous humour of the posterior chamber of the eye.
Atherogenic	Any process stimulating the production of atheroma, a substance laid down in the wall of the blood vessel and tending to obstruct it.
Atherosclerotic	A group of pathological conditions causing narrowing of the blood vessels. 'Hardening of the arteries.'
Atrophic	Wasting.
Autoimmune	The production of antibodies to body tissues by the body.
Autonomic	That part of the nervous system (parasympathetic and sympathetic)

responsible for the automatic regulation of bodily functions.

Axon/axonal — Part of a nerve cell.

Axoplasm — The cytoplasm within the nerve cell.

B

Bacteroides — A group of bacteria causing infection.

Balanitis — An inflammation of the foreskin.

Biosthesiometer — A simple machine which consists of an electronic tuning fork which vibrates at a fixed frequency and at an amplitude (and therefore intensity) which is proportional to the voltage applied to the tuning fork. A volt meter is included in the circuit which therefore provides a means of assessing the intensity of the vibration. By increasing or decreasing the voltage the intensity of vibration can be varied and the machine used to assess the vibration threshold.

Bipolar cells — Nerve cells having two main processes (axons).

Bruit — Murmur, the sound of turbulent blood flow heard with the aid of a stethoscope.

C

Cardiorespiratory — Referring to heart and lungs.

Carotid endarterectomy — A surgical procedure which consists of removing the diseased lining of the carotid artery.

Catecholamines — A group of chemical substances (adrenaline and adrenaline like) produced by the adrenal gland.

Choriocapillaris — A fine layer of capillaries beneath the choroid layer of the eye.

Claudication — Usually used to indicate pain in the leg on walking caused by insufficient blood reaching the muscles. (e.g. when blood vessels are severely narrowed).

Clostridium perfringens — A bacterium causing infection.

Cortisol	Cortisone – a chemical substance (hormone) produced by the adrenal cortex.

D

Demographic data	Statistics relating to the structure of a population, e.g. in terms of age, sex and race.
Demyelination	The loss of the myelin covering of nerve fibres which causes them to malfunction.
Dendrites	Short processes of a nerve cell which enables it to receive communications from another nerve cell.
Diuresis	Abnormally great excretion of urine.
Doppler	Christiana Doppler was an Austrian mathematician (1803–1853). He described the effect of movement on frequency. Thus the pitch of a whistle on a locomotive or other rapidly moving body is higher when the machine is approaching the listener and lower as it moves away. The principle is used for measuring blood flow. A beam of sound is passed into a blood vessel and is reflected back by the red cells contained therein. The movement of the red cells alters the frequency of the sound and the change in frequency may be detected by a suitable electronic apparatus. The change in frequency is proportional to the rate of flow and this change may be either displayed as a sound (the Doppler stethoscope) or as numerical data.
Dystrophic	Poorly nourished.

E

Encephalopathy	A disorder of the brain.
Endothelial	The lining of blood vessels.

F

Fluoroscein angiography	A means of outlining blood vessels in the eye by injecting a fluorescent dye and using a suitably arranged photographic apparatus.
Funduscopy	The examination of the retina using an ophthalmoscope.

G

Gastroparesis	A paralysis of the muscles of the stomach producing gastric dilatation.
Glomerulosclerosis	Progressive destruction of glomeruli and replacement by fibrous tissue.
Glomerulus	The knot of capillaries in the kidney which act as a filter.
Gluconeogenesis	The production of glucose by the liver from other molecules.
Glycaemic control	Relating to the maintenance of blood glucose levels within normal limits.
Glycogenolysis	The production of glucose from glycogen by the liver.
Glycolytic pathway	The series of chemical reactions describing the break down of glucose.
Glycosylated haemoglobin	Haemoglobin that has been altered by a chemical reaction with glucose.
Gustatory	Relating to taste.

H

Haematocrit	The proportion of solid elements (e.g. red cells and white cells) in the blood.
Hallux rigidus	A condition in which walking is painful on account of stiffness in the metatarsophalangeal joint of the great toe.
Harris mat	A simple apparatus used for measuring pressure areas on the lower surfaces of the feet.
Heparinized	Treated with heparin (an anticoagulant).

Histocompatibility antigens	Antigens which are expressed on the surface of cells and which are genetically controlled. They are used in tissue typing which has been found useful in transplantation. The presence of these antigens may be associated with an increased susceptibility to certain disorders.
Homeostasis	The process through which bodily chemical and physical equilibrium is maintained.
Hyperbilirubinaemia	An increased amount of bile in the blood.
Hyperlipidaemia	An increased amount of fat in the blood.
Hypermetropia	Long sight
Hypernatraemia	An increased amount of sodium in the blood.
Hyperosmolar	A high concentration of small molecules in the blood giving rise to a high osmolarity.
Hyperuricaemia	An increased amount of urate (uric acid) in the blood.
Hypocalcaemia	A decreased amount of calcium in the blood.
Hypokalaemia	A decrease in the concentration of potassium in the blood.
Hypotension	A blood pressure lower than normal.
Hypovolaemia	A diminished blood volume.

I

Intertrigo	Dermatitis resulting from infection of the skin where skin folds come into contact, e.g. beneath the breasts.
Ischaemia	A lack of blood.
Isotopic bone scan	A means of assessing abnormalities in bone using radioactive isotopes.

K

Ketoacidosis	Excessive quantities of acid in the blood due to the presence of substances called

	ketoacids. These substances are produced when there is a lack of insulin which normally inhibits their production.
Ketosis	An excessive quantity of ketones in the blood.
Kimmelstiel-Wilson syndrome	Kimmelstiel and Wilson described a histological picture seen in patients suffering from diabetic kidney disease. Nodular glomerular sclerosis.

L

Lacticacidosis	An excessive quantity of acid in the blood due to the presence of lactic acid.
Laser Doppler flowmetry	A technique for measuring the blood flow in small vessels using the Doppler principle and utilizing the properties of laser light.
Lipaemia retinalis	An appearance seen in the retina due to excessive quantities of fat in the blood.
Loop of Henle	The nephron is the functional unit of the kidney. It consists of a knot of capillaries, the glomerulus which leads to a convoluted tube (the proximal convoluted tubule). This leads to a U-shaped long looped tube known as the loop of Henle which in turn leads to the distal convoluted tubule and then on to the collecting ducts. During its passage through this tubular system the glomerular filtrate is converted to urine.

M

Macroalbuminuria	A quantity of albumin present in the urine detectable by the use of a dip-stick such as Albustix.
Macrovascular disease	Disease of large blood vessels.
Macula	That area of the retina which is sensitive to high-intensity light and colour. It is

	the area responsible for detailed vision.
Mesangium	Part of the glomerulus.
Microalbuminuria	The presence of abnormal amounts of albumin in the urine but not sufficient to be detectable by simple dip stick such as Albustix (see macroalbuminuria).
Microvascular disease	Disease of small vessels.
Mononeuritis	Inflammation of a single nerve.
Mononeuritis multiplex	Inflammation of several unrelated nerves.
Mydriatic	A substance used for dilating the pupil.
Myelin	The substance which ensheathes the axons of certain nerve fibres.
Myocardial infarction	Death of heart muscle due to a reduced blood supply, usually resulting from coronary artery disease.
Myopia	Short sight.

N

Necrobiosis lipoidica diabeticorum	A skin condition seen in diabetes. It most commonly occurs on the front of the lower legs but may appear on the upper limbs or trunk. It usually starts with raised red papules with a yellowish middle which slowly coalesce and spread. The centre becomes atrophic (necrobiosis) and is associated with a deposition of yellowish material of fatty origin (lipoidica).
Neovascularization	The production of new vessels in the retina. The revascularization of ischaemic retina.
Nephron	The functional unit of the kidney (see also glomerulus and loop of Henle.
Neurogenic	Symptoms mediated through the activities of the nervous system.
Neuroglycopenia	The effect caused by a low blood glucose on the brain.
Neuropathy	Disease of nerves.

Nocturia	The necessity to pass urine in the night.
Normoalbuminuria	The presence of albumin in the urine within the accepted normal limits.

O

Oliguric	The production of a volume of urine below that which is considered normal.

P

Papillary necrosis	Destruction of that part of the kidney known as the renal papilla.
Paraesthesia	'Pins and needles'.
PCO_2, PO_2	The partial pressure of carbon dioxide or oxygen in the blood.
Percutaneous transluminal angioplasty	A means of opening narrowed blood vessels by passing a tube through the skin (per cutaneous) into the lumen of a blood vessel (transluminal) and expanding a balloon in the narrowed area of the blood vessel (angioplasty) and thus dilating it.
Pericytes	Small cells situated in the wall of blood vessels supplying the retina.
Peripheral vascular disease	Disease of blood vessels supplying the peripheral part of the body.
Photocoagulation	A means of destroying tissues by the use of high-intensity light beams.
Polydipsia	Excessive thirst.
Polymyalgia	A condition characterized by muscle pain.
Polyuria	Passing of excessive quantities of urine.
Popliteal	Referring to the area behind the knee.
Prophylactic	Preventative.
Pruritus vulvae	Symptoms of itching in the vulva.
Pupillomotor	The nerve fibres which actuate the mechanism of constriction and dilatation of the pupil.

R

Retinopathy	Disease of the retina.

Retrohyaloid haemorrhage	Haemorrhage between the vitreous body in the posterior chamber of the eye and the retina.
Rubeotic glaucoma	Raised internal pressure in the eye due to invasion of the filtration angle by new vessels.

S

Saucerize	To open out an ulcer to assist drainage.
Sequestrate	To hide away.
Sine qua non	Requirement.
Solute	A substance dissolved in a solvent to produce a solution

T

Tented T waves	The shape of the T wave on the ECG indicating excessive concentrations of potassium in the blood.
Thromboses	The obstruction of blood vessels by the formation of clot.
Tinea pedis	Athletes foot. A fungal infection.
Toxoplasma	A parasitic infection.
Transcutaneous oximetry	A means of measuring the amount of oxygen in and beneath the skin using a transducer placed over the skin.
Transluminal angioplasty	See percutaneous transluminal angioplasty

U

Uraemic	An excessive quantity of urea in the blood.

V

Vasa nervorum	The small blood vessels which supply nerves.
Vibration sense	The ability to feel a vibrating tuning fork when it is placed on a bony prominence in any part of the body.

W

Whitfield's Ointment	Compound benzoic acid ointment used in the local treatment of fungal infections.
WHO	World Health Organization.

X

Xanthelasma	Deposits of fatty substance under the skin giving rise to yellowish streaks around the eyelids.

Index